This report contains the collective views of an international group of experts and does not necessarily represent the decisions or the stated policy of the United Nations Environment Programme, the International Labour Organisation, or the World Health Organization

Environmental Health Criteria 99

CYHALOTHRIN

Published under the joint sponsorship of the United Nations Environment Programme, the International Labour Organisation, and the World Health Organization

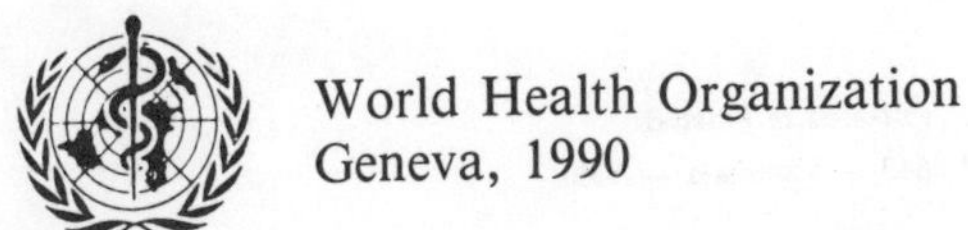

World Health Organization
Geneva, 1990

The **International Programme on Chemical Safety (IPCS)** is a joint venture of the United Nations Environment Programme, the International Labour Organisation, and the World Health Organization. The main objective of the IPCS is to carry out and disseminate evaluations of the effects of chemicals on human health and the quality of the environment. Supporting activities include the development of epidemiological, experimental laboratory, and risk-assessment methods that could produce internationally comparable results, and the development of manpower in the field of toxicology. Other activities carried out by the IPCS include the development of know-how for coping with chemical accidents, coordination of laboratory testing and epidemiological studies, and promotion of research on the mechanisms of the biological action of chemicals.

WHO Library Cataloguing in Publication Data

Cyhalothrin.

(Environmental health criteria ; 99)

1.Pyrethrins - adverse effects 2.Pyrethrins - toxicity I.Series

ISBN 92 4 154299 3 (NLM Classification: WA 240)
ISSN 0250-863X

The designations employed and the presentation of the material in this publication do not imply the expression of any opinion whatsoever on the part of the Secretariat of the World Health Organization concerning the legal status of any country, territory, city, or area or of its authorities, or concerning the delimitation of its frontiers or boundaries.

The mention of specific companies or of certain manufacturers' products does not imply that they are endorsed or recommended by the World Health Organization in preference to others of a similar nature that are not mentioned. Errors and omissions excepted, the names of proprietary products are distinguished by initial capital letters.

Printed in Finland
90/8643 — Vammala — 5000

CONTENTS

WHO TASK GROUP ON ENVIRONMENTAL HEALTH CRITERIA FOR CYHALOTHRIN

Members

Dr V. Benes, Toxicology and Reference Laboratory, Institute of Hygiene and Epidemiology, Prague, Czechoslovakia

Dr A.J. Browning, Toxicology Evaluation Section, Department of Community Services and Health, Woden, ACT, Australia

Dr S. Dobson, Institute of Terrestrial Ecology, Monks Wood Experimental Station, Abbots Ripton, Huntingdon, United Kingdom (*Chairman*)

Dr P. Hurley, Office of Pesticide Programme, US Environmental Protection Agency, Washington, DC, USA

Dr K. Imaida, Section of Tumour Pathology, Division of Pathology, National Institute of Hygienic Sciences, Setagaya-Ku, Tokyo, Japan

Dr S.K. Kashyap, National Institute of Occupational Health, (I.C.M.R.) Ahmedabad, India (*Vice-Chairman*)

Dr Yu. I. Kundiev, Research Institute of Labour, Hygiene and Occupational Diseases, Ul. Saksaganskogo, Kiev, USSR

Dr J.P. Leahey, ICI Agrochemicals, Jealotts Hill Research Station, Bracknell, United Kingdom (*Joint Rapporteur*)

Dr M. Matsuo, Sumitomo Chemical Company, Biochemistry and Toxicology Laboratory, Kasugade-naka, Konohana-Ku, Osaka, Japan

Representatives of Other Organizations

Mr M. L'Hotellier, International Group of National Associations of Manufacturers of Agricultural Products (GIFAP)

Dr N. Punja, International Group of National Associations of Manufacturers of Agricultural Products (GIFAP)

Secretariat

Dr K.W. Jager, International Programme on Chemical Safety, World Health Organization, Geneva, Switzerland (*Secretary*)

Dr R. Plestina, Division of Vector Biology and Control, World Health Organization, Geneva, Switzerland

Dr J. Sekizawa, Division of Information on Chemical Safety, National Institute of Hygienic Sciences, Setagaya-Ku, Tokyo, Japan (*Joint Rapporteur*)

NOTE TO READERS OF THE CRITERIA DOCUMENTS

Every effort has been made to present information in the criteria documents as accurately as possible without unduly delaying their publication. In the interest of all users of the environmental health criteria documents, readers are kindly requested to communicate any errors that may have occurred to the Manager of the International Programme on Chemical Safety, World Health Organization, Geneva, Switzerland, in order that they may be included in corrigenda, which will appear in subsequent volumes.

* * *

A detailed data profile and a legal file can be obtained from the International Register of Potentially Toxic Chemicals, Palais des Nations, 1211 Geneva 10, Switzerland (Telephone No. 7988400 or 7985850).

* * *

The proprietary information contained in this document cannot replace documentation for registration purposes, because the latter has to be closely linked to the source, the manufacturing route, and the purity/impurities of the substance to be registered. The data should be used in accordance with paragraphs 82-84 and recommendations paragraph 90 of the Second FAO Government Consultation (1982).

ENVIRONMENTAL HEALTH CRITERIA FOR CYHALOTHRIN

A WHO Task Group meeting on Environmental Health Criteria for Cyhalothrin was held in Geneva from 24 to 28 October 1988. Dr M. Mercier, Manager, IPCS, opened the meeting and welcomed the participants on behalf of the three IPCS cooperating organizations (UNEP/ILO/WHO). The group reviewed and revised the draft monograph and made an evaluation of the risks for human health and the environment from exposure to cyhalothrin.

The first draft was prepared by the IPCS Secretariat based on material made available by ICI Agrochemicals, United Kingdom.

The second draft was also prepared by the IPCS Secretariat, incorporating comments received following circulation of the first draft to the IPCS contact points for Environmental Health Criteria monographs. Dr K.W. Jager and Dr P.G. Jenkins, both members of the IPCS Central Unit, were responsible for the technical development and editing, respectively, of this monograph.

The assistance of ICI Agrochemicals in making available to the IPCS and the Task Group its toxicological proprietary information on cyhalothrin is gratefully acknowledged. This allowed the Task Group to make its evaluation on the basis of more complete data.

ABBREVIATIONS

ADI	acceptable daily intake
ai	active ingredient
APDM	aminopyrine-*N*-demethylase
EC	emulsifiable concentrate
ECD	electron capture detection
GC	gas chromatography
HPLC	high performance liquid chromatography
LOEL	lowest-observed-effect level
MS	mass spectrometry
MSD	mass selective detection
NOEL	no-observed-effect-level
SFS	subjective facial sensation
TLC	thin-layer chromatography
WP	wettable powder

INTRODUCTION

SYNTHETIC PYRETHROIDS - A PROFILE

1. During investigations to modify the chemical structures of natural pyrethrins, a certain number of synthetic pyrethroids were produced with improved physical and chemical properties and greater biological activity. Several of the earlier synthetic pyrethroids were successfully commercialized, mainly for the control of household insects. Other more recent pyrethroids have been introduced as agricultural insecticides because of their excellent activity against a wide range of insect pests and their non-persistence in the environment.

2. The pyrethroids constitute another group of insecticides in addition to organochlorine, organophosphorus, carbamate, and other compounds. Pyrethroids commercially available to date include allethrin, resmethrin, d-phenothrin, and tetramethrin (for insects of public health importance), and cypermethrin, deltamethrin, fenvalerate, and permethrin (mainly for agricultural insects). Other pyrethroids are also available including furamethrin, kadethrin, and tellallethrin (usually for household insects), fenpropathrin, tralomethrin, cyhalothrin, lambda-cyhalothrin, tefluthrin, cyfluthrin, flucythrinate, fluvalinate, and biphenate (for agricultural insects).

3. Toxicological evaluations of several synthetic pyrethroids have been performed by the FAO/WHO Joint Meeting on Pesticide Residues (JMPR). The acceptable daily intake (ADI) has been estimated by the JMPR for cypermethrin, deltamethrin, fenvalerate, permethrin, d-phenothrin, cyfluthrin, cyhalothrin, and flucythrinate.

4. Chemically, synthetic pyrethroids are esters of specific acids (e.g., chrysanthemic acid, halo-substituted chrysanthemic acid, 2-(4-chlorophenyl)-3-methylbutyric acid) and alcohols (e.g., allethrolone, 3-phenoxybenzyl alcohol). For certain pyrethroids, the asymmetric centre(s) exist in the acid and/or alcohol moiety, and the commercial products sometimes consist of a mixture of both optical (1R/1S or d/1) and geometric (cis/trans) isomers. However, most

of the insecticidal activity of such products may reside in only one or two isomers. Some of the products (e.g., d-phenothrin, deltamethrin) consist only of such active isomer(s).

5. Synthetic pyrethroids are neuropoisons acting on the axons in the peripheral and central nervous systems by interacting with sodium channels in mammals and/or insects. A single dose produces toxic signs in mammals, such as tremors, hyperexcitability, salivation, choreoathetosis, and paralysis. The signs disappear fairly rapidly, and the animals recover, generally within a week. At near-lethal dose levels, synthetic pyrethroids cause transient changes in the nervous system, such as axonal swelling and/or breaks and myelin degeneration in sciatic nerves. They are not considered to cause delayed neurotoxicity of the kind induced by some organophosphorus compounds. The mechanism of toxicity of synthetic pyrethroids and their classification into two types are discussed in the Appendix.

6. Some pyrethroids (e.g., deltamethrin, fenvalerate, cyhalothrin, lambda-cyhalothrin, flucythrinate, and cypermethrin) may cause a transient itching and/or burning sensation in exposed human skin.

7. Synthetic pyrethroids are generally metabolized in mammals through ester hydrolysis, oxidation, and conjugation, and there is no tendency to accumulate in tissues. In the environment, synthetic pyrethroids are fairly rapidly degraded in soil and in plants. Ester hydrolysis and oxidation at various sites on the molecule are the major degradation processes. The pyrethroids are strongly adsorbed on soil and sediments, and hardly eluted with water. There is little tendency for bioaccumulation in organisms.

8. Because of low application rates and rapid degradation in the environment, residues in food are generally low.

9. Synthetic pyrethroids have been shown to be toxic for fish, aquatic arthropods, and honey-bees in laboratory tests. But, in practical usage, no serious adverse effects have been noticed because of the low rates of application and lack of persistence in the environment. The toxicity of synthetic pyrethroids in birds and domestic animals is low.

10. In addition to the evaluation documents of FAO/WHO, there are several good reviews and books on the chemistry, metabolism, mammalian toxicity, environmental effects, etc., of synthetic pyrethroids, including those by Elliott (1977), Miyamoto (1981), Miyamoto & Kearney (1983), and Leahey (1985).

1. SUMMARY, EVALUATION, CONCLUSIONS, AND RECOMMENDATIONS

1.1 Summary and evaluation

1.1.1 Identity, physical and chemical properties, analytical methods

Cyhalothrin is formed by esterifying 3-(2-chloro-3,3,3-trifluoroprop-1-enyl)-2,2-dimethylcyclopropanecarboxylic acid with α-cyano-3-phenoxybenzyl alcohol, and it consists of a mixture of four stereoisomers. Lambda-cyhalothrin consists of one enantiomeric pair of isomers and is the more biologically active form.

Technical grade cyhalothrin is a yellow-brown viscous liquid (melting point: approximately 10 °C) and contains more than 90% active material. It is composed of four cis isomers in the ratio of 1:1:1:1. Although it is insoluble in water, it is soluble in a range of organic solvents such as aliphatic and aromatic hydrocarbons. It is stable to light and heat and has a low vapour pressure.

Technical grade lambda-cyhalothrin is a beige solid (melting point: 49.2 °C) and contains more than 90% active material. The enantiomer ratio of the (*Z*), (*1R*, *3R*), S-ester to the (*Z*), (*1S*, *3S*), R-ester is 1:1. It is sparingly soluble in water but soluble in a range of organic solvents and has a low vapour pressure. Both cyhalothrin and lambda-cyhalothrin are rapidly hydrolysed under alkaline conditions but not in neutral or acidic media.

Well established methods for residue and environmental analysis of cyhalothrin and lambda-cyhalothrin are available (the minimum detectable concentration is 0.005 mg/kg).

1.1.2 Production and use

Cyhalothrin was developed in 1977. It is principally used to combat a wide range of pests in public health and animal health, but is also employed in agriculture against pests of pome fruit. Lambda-cyhalothrin is mainly used as an agricultural pesticide on a wide range of crops and is being developed for public health.

No data are available on production levels.

1.1.3 Human exposure

Residues in food arising from the use of cyhalothrin and lambda-cyhalothrin on crops and in animal health are low, usually less than 0.2 mg/kg. No results are available on the total dietary intake in humans, but it can be assumed that the dietary exposure of the general population will not exceed the ADI (0.02 mg/kg body weight).

1.1.4 Environmental exposure and fate

On soil surfaces and in aqueous solutions at pH 5, lambda-cyhalothrin degrades in sunlight with a half-life of approximately 30 days. The main degradation products are 3-(2-chloro-3,3,3-trifluoroprop-1-enyl)-2,2-dimethylcyclopropanecarboxylic acid, the amide derivative of cyhalothrin, and 3-phenoxybenzoic acid.

Degradation in soil occurs primarily by hydroxylation followed by cleavage of the ester linkage to give two main degradation products, which are further degraded to carbon dioxide. The initial half-lives are in the range of 22 to 82 days.

Cyhalothrin and lambda-cyhalothrin are adsorbed on soil particles and are non-mobile in the environment.

On plants lambda-cyhalothrin degrades at a moderate rate (half-life of up to 40 days), so that the major constituent of the residue on plants is usually the parent compound. Lower levels of metabolites, resulting from a range of hydrolytic and oxidative reactions, are also found.

No data are available on actual levels in the environment, but with the low current use pattern and low application rates, these are expected to be low.

1.1.5 Uptake, metabolism, and excretion

Metabolic studies have been carried out on the rat, dog, cow, and goat. In rats and dogs, cyhalothrin has been shown to be well absorbed after oral administration, extensively metabolized, and eliminated as polar conjugates in urine. Cyhalothrin levels in rat tissues declined upon cessation of exposure to the compound. Residues in rat carcasses were low (< 5% of the dose after 7 days) and were found to be almost entirely due to cyhalothrin contained in fats. Residues in fats were eliminated with a half-life of 23 days.

After oral administration to lactating cows, cyhalothrin was rapidly eliminated, an equilibrium between ingestion and elimination being reached after 3 days. Of the overall dose, 27% was excreted in the urine, 50% in the faeces, and 0.8% in the milk. Urinary material consisted entirely of ester cleavage metabolites and their conjugates, whereas 60-70% of the faecal [^{14}C]-labelled material was identified as unchanged cyhalothrin. Tissue residues, 16 h after the last dose, were low, the highest concentrations being detected in fat. The [^{14}C]-labelled residues in milk and fatty tissues were almost entirely unchanged cyhalothrin, no other component being detected.

In all mammalian species investigated, cyhalothrin has been found to be extensively metabolized as a result of ester cleavage to the cyclopropanecarboxylic acid and 3-phenoxybenzoic acid, and eliminated as conjugates.

In fish the main residue in tissues consists of unchanged cyhalothrin, and there are lower levels of the ester cleavage products.

1.1.6 Effects on organisms in the environment

Under laboratory conditions of constant toxicant concentrations, cyhalothrin and lambda-cyhalothrin are highly toxic to fish and to aquatic invertebrates. The 96-h LC_{50} values for fish range between 0.2 and 1.3 μg/litre, whereas for aquatic invertebrates the 48-h LC_{50} values range between 0.008 and 0.4 μg/litre.

Accumulation studies conducted under laboratory conditions with constant concentration show that rapid uptake takes place in fish (accumulation factor approximately 1000-2000). However, in the presence of soil and suspended sediment, the bioaccumulation factors are greatly reduced (to 19 in the case of fish and 194 in the case of daphnids). When exposed fish and daphnids were placed in clean water the residues declined rapidly, with half-lives of 7 days and 1 day, respectively. The concentrations of cyhalothrin and lambda-cyhalothrin that are likely to arise in water from normal agricultural application will be low. Since the compound is rapidly adsorbed and degraded under natural conditions, there will not be any practical problems concerning the accumulation of residues or the toxicity of cyhalothrin or lambda-cyhalothrin in aquatic species.

Cyhalothrin and lambda-cyhalothrin are virtually non-toxic to birds; the single-dose LD_{50} was greater than 3950 mg/kg in all species tested and the lowest 5-day dietary LC_{50} was 3948 mg/kg (lambda-cyhalothrin fed to 8-day-old mallard ducks).

Under laboratory conditions, cyhalothrin and lambda-cyhalothrin are toxic to honey-bees; the oral LD_{50} for lambda-cyhalothrin is 0.97 μg/bee. However, in the field the hazard is lower since current formulations have a repellant action that causes a suspension of foraging activity in treated crops. When foraging restarts there is no significant increase in bee mortality.

1.1.7 Effects on experimental animals and in vitro test systems

The acute oral toxicity of cyhalothrin is moderate in rats and mice and low in guinea-pigs and rabbits (LD_{50} values are as follows: rat, 144-243 mg/kg; mouse, 37-62 mg/kg; guinea-pig, > 5000 mg/kg; rabbit, > 1000 mg/kg). The acute oral toxicity of lambda-cyhalothrin is higher than that of cyhalothrin (LD_{50} values are: 56-79 mg/kg for the rat and 20 mg/kg for the mouse). The dermal toxicities (LD_{50}) are as follows: rat, 200-2000 mg/kg (cyhalothrin), 632-696 mg/kg (lambda-cyhalothrin); rabbit, > 2000 mg/kg (cyhalothrin). Cyhalothrin and lambda-cyhalothrin are type II pyrethroids; clinical signs include ataxia, unsteady gait, and hyperexcitability.

In the rabbit, cyhalothrin is a moderate eye irritant and lambda-cyhalothrin is a mild eye irritant; both are mild skin irritants. Cyhalothrin is not a skin irritant in the rat. However, it is a moderate skin sensitizer in the guinea-pig. Lambda-cyhalothrin is not a skin sensitizer.

In a 90-day feeding study in which rats were fed cyhalothrin at dose levels up to 250 mg/kg diet, reduced body weight gains were observed in males at 250 mg/kg diet. Marginal effects on mean erythrocyte volumes were noted in some treated groups, as well as some liver changes, which were considered to be an adaptive response. In a 90-day feeding study in which rats were fed lambda-cyhalothrin at dose levels up to 250 mg/kg diet, reduced body weight gain was observed in both sexes at 250 mg/kg diet. Some effects on clinical chemistry were observed, as well as liver effects similar to those noted with cyhalothrin. The no-observed-effect level was 50 mg/kg diet.

In a 26-week oral study in which cyhalothrin doses of up to 10 mg/kg body weight per day were administered to dogs, signs of pyrethroid toxicity were observed at 10 mg per kg body weight per day. The no-observed-effect level was 2.5 mg/kg body weight per day. A similar study was conducted in which up to 3.5 mg lambda-cyhalothrin/kg body weight per day was administered to dogs for 52 weeks. Clinical signs of pyrethroid toxicity (neurological signs) were observed in all animals dosed with 3.5 mg/kg body weight per day. The no-observed-effect level was 0.5 mg/kg body weight per day.

In a 21-day dermal study on rabbits using cyhalothrin in polyethylene glycol at dose levels of up to 1000 mg/kg per day, clinical signs of toxicity were observed in some animals at the highest dose level. Slight to severe skin irritation was observed in all groups, including controls.

Cyhalothrin was tested in two 104-week feeding studies, one on rats and one on mice. In the rat study, no oncogenic effects were observed at dose levels up to 250 mg/kg diet (highest level tested). The no-observed-effect level for systemic toxicity was 50 mg/kg diet (1.8 mg/kg body weight per day). Decreased body weight gain was observed in both sexes at 250 mg/kg diet. In the mouse study, no oncogenic effects were observed at dose levels up to 500 mg/kg diet (highest level tested). Clinical signs of pyrethroid toxicity were observed at 100 and 500 mg/kg diet, and reduced body weight gain was observed at 500 mg/kg diet. The no-observed-effect level for systemic toxicity was 20 mg/kg diet (1.9 mg/kg body weight per day). No histological evidence of damage to the nervous system was observed in either study.

Cyhalothrin and lambda-cyhalothrin gave negative results in a range of *in vivo* and *in vitro* assays designed to detect gene mutations, chromosomal damage, and other genotoxic effects. When orally administered to the rat and rabbit during the period of major organogenesis, cyhalothrin was neither embryotoxic nor teratogenic at dose levels that elicited maternal toxicity (15 mg/kg per day for rats and 30 mg/kg per day for rabbits, both highest dose levels tested).

A three-generation reproduction study was conducted on rats with cyhalothrin at dose levels of up to 100 mg/kg diet. Minor decreases in litter size and small reductions in weight gain were seen at 100 mg/kg diet. The no-observed-effect level for reproductive effects was 30 mg per kg diet.

1.1.8 Effects on humans

No cases of accidental poisoning have been described.

In manufacturing, formulation, laboratory work, and field usage, symptoms of subjective facial sensation have been reported. This effect generally lasts only a few hours, but occasionally persists for up to 72 h after exposure; medical examination has not revealed any neurological abnormalities.

Subjective facial skin sensations, which may be experienced by people who handle cyhalothrin and lambda-cyhalothrin, are believed to be brought about by repetitive firing of sensory nerve terminals in the skin. They may be considered as an early warning signal indicating that overexposure of the skin has occurred.

There are no indications that cyhalothrin and lambda-cyhalothrin, used under the present recommended conditions and application rates, will have any adverse effect on humans.

1.2 Conclusions

(a) *General population:* The exposure of the general population to cyhalothrin and lambda-cyhalothrin is expected to be very low and is not likely to present a hazard under recommended conditions of use.

(b) *Occupational exposure:* With good work practices, hygiene measures, and safety precautions, cyhalothrin and lambda-cyhalothrin are unlikely to present a hazard to those occupationally exposed.

(c) *Environment:* It is unlikely that cyhalothrin and lambda-cyhalothrin or their degradation products will attain levels of adverse environmental significance with recommended application rates. Under laboratory conditions cyhalothrin and lambda-cyhalothrin are highly toxic to fish, aquatic arthropods, and honey-bees. However, under field conditions, lasting adverse effects are not likely to occur under recommended conditions of use.

1.3 Recommendations

Although dietary levels from recommended usage are considered to be very low, confirmation of this through inclusion of cyhalothrin and lambda-cyhalothrin in monitoring studies should be considered.

Although cyhalothrin and lambda-cyhalothrin have been used for several years and any effects from occupational exposure have been only transient, observations of human exposure should be maintained.

2. IDENTITY, PHYSICAL AND CHEMICAL PROPERTIES, ANALYTICAL METHODS

2.1 Identity

Molecular formula: $C_{23}H_{19}ClF_3NO_3$

Chemical structure:

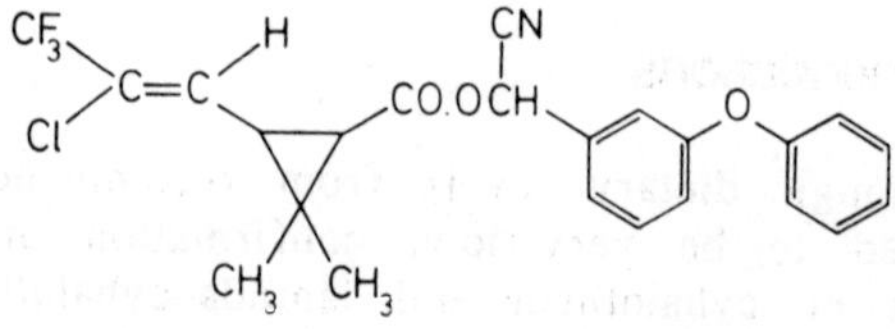

Chemical name:	α-cyano-3-phenoxybenzyl 3-(2-chloro-3,3,3-trifluoroprop-1-enyl)-2,2-dimethyl-cyclopropanecarboxylate
CAS Chemical name:	(*RS*)-α-cyano-3-(phenoxyphenyl)methyl (*1RS*)-*cis*-3-(*Z*-2-chloro-3,3,3-tri-fluoroprop-1-enyl)-2,2-dimethylcyclopro-panecarboxylate
CAS registry: number	cyhalothrin: 68085-85-8 lambda-cyhalothrin: 91465-08-6
Common synonyms:	cyhalothrin: R114563, PP563 lambda-cyhalothrin: R119321, PP321
Trade names:	cyhalothrin: Grenade lambda-cyhalothrin: Karate, Matador, Icon

Cyhalothrin was developed by ICI in 1977. It is prepared by esterification of 3-(2-chloro-3,3,3-trifluoroprop-1-enyl)-2,2-dimethylcyclopropanecarboxylic acid chloride with α-cyano-3-phenoxybenzyl alcohol.

Cyhalothrin has two asymmetric centres in the acid moiety and one in the alcohol moiety, as well as Z and E

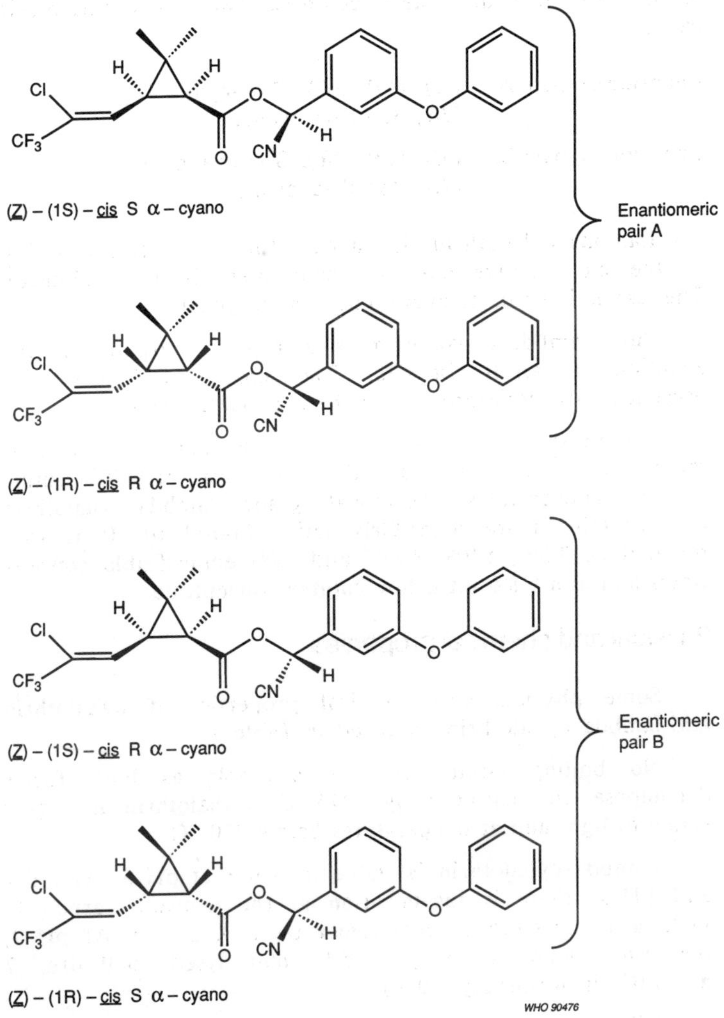

Cl CF3 H H O O CN H O
(Z) – (1S) – cis S α – cyano

Cl CF3 H H O O CN H O
(Z) – (1R) – cis R α – cyano

Enantiomeric pair A

Cl CF3 H H O O CN H O
(Z) – (1S) – cis R α – cyano

Cl CF3 H H O O CN H O
(Z) – (1R) – cis S α – cyano

Enantiomeric pair B

WHO 90476

Fig. 1. Chemical structures of the two enantiomeric pairs of isomers comprising cyhalothrin.

forms. Thus, there are 16 possible isomeric forms (eight enantiomeric pairs). However, in practice cyhalothrin is produced only in the Z and cis forms, reducing the number of isomers to four. These comprise two cis enantiomeric pairs:

Enantiomer pair A: (*Z*), (*1R*, *3R*), R-α-cyano (*Z*), (*1S*, *3S*) S-α-cyano;

Enantiomer pair B: (*Z*), (*1R*, *3R*), S-α-cyano (*Z*), (*1S*, *3S*) R-α-cyano.

Lambda-cyhalothrin is manufactured by crystallization of the more active pair of enantiomers from cyhalothrin. The less active pair of enantiomers is recycled.

Pure lambda-cyhalothrin is a racemic mixture of the enantiomer pair B isomers. The enantiomer pair A is present in low concentration in the commercial product.

Technical grade cyhalothrin contains more than 90% of the pesticide and is formulated in 5%, 10%, and 20% emulsifiable concentrates. Technical grade lambda-cyhalothrin also contains more than 90% active ingredient. It is formulated as 2.5%, 5.0%, 8.3%, and 12% emulsifiable concentrates and as a 0.8% ultra-low volume concentrate.

2.2 Physical and chemical properties

Some physical and chemical properties of cyhalothrin and lambda-cyhalothrin are listed in Table 1.

No boiling point data are available as both forms decompose on heating above 275 °C. Cyhalothrin is highly stable to light and at temperatures below 220 °C.

Lambda-cyhalothrin is stable in water at pH 5. At pH 7 and pH 9, there is racemization at the α-cyano carbon to yield a 1:1 mixture of enantiomer pairs A and B. At pH 9, the ester bond is fairly readily hydrolysed (half-life, 7 days) (Collis & Leahey, 1984).

Dilute aqueous solutions are subject to photolysis at a moderate rate (Hall & Leahey, 1983; Curl et al., 1984a).

2.3 Analytical methods

The most widely adopted procedures for analysing cyhalothrin residues in crops, soil, animal tissues and

Table 1. Some physical and chemical properties of cyhalothrin and lambda-cyhalothrin

	Cyhalothrin	Lambda-cyhalothrin
Physical state	viscous liquid	solid
Colour	yellow-brown	beige
Odour	mild	mild
Relative molecular mass	449.9	449.9
Melting point	glass-like below 10 °C	49.2 °C
Decomposes	> 275 °C	> 275 °C
Water solubility	4×10^{-3} mg/litre	5×10^{-3} mg/litre
Solubility in organic solvents	soluble	soluble
n-octanol water-partition coefficient (log P_{ow}) at 20 °C	6.9	7.0
Relative density	1.25	1.33
Vapour pressure at 20 °C	1×10^{-9} kPa	2×10^{-10} kPa
Vapour pressure at 80 °C	4×10^{-6} kPa	3×10^{-6} kPa

products, and environmental samples are based on extraction of the residue with organic solvent, clean-up of the extract by solvent-solvent partition and adsorption column chromatography, and determination of the residue using gas chromatography (GC) with electron capture detection (GC/ECD). The identity of residues can be confirmed by GC with mass selective detection (GC-MSD) or by thin-layer chromatography (TLC) followed by GC/ECD.

2.3.1 *Sampling methods*

Procedures for obtaining representative samples of crops, processed commodities, soil, and some animal products have been described in detail (GIFAP, 1981) and will not be discussed further.

Particular care is necessary when sampling water because cyhalothrin is extremely hydrophobic and rapidly adsorbs onto particulates or container walls from aqueous solution. For this reason, the whole analytical sample should be taken for analysis and not subdivided in the field (Sapiets et al., 1984). Collection of the sample in a clean glass container, with addition of the extraction solvent before sealing and shaking the bottle, gives good recoveries. Crossland et al. (1982) described procedures for sampling surface water (using stainless steel fine mesh discs) and subsurface water from ponds for separate analysis of cypermethrin. Precautions were taken to avoid contamination during sampling (Crossland et al., 1982). These methods, developed for cypermethrin, are equally applicable to cyhalothrin and other pyrethroids. During the course of the pond studies, cypermethrin spray drift deposits were collected by means of horizontally placed aluminium foil plates and washed from the foils using acetone. Crossland also described the use of a core sampler to remove pond sediment for cypermethrin analysis (Crossland, 1982). This method is equally applicable to cyhalothrin.

Sampling of air in agriculture work space for pyrethroid aerosol droplets using absorption onto exposed filter papers and porous glass slides has been described by Girenko & Klisenko (1984). They quoted limits in the range of 0.05 to 0.5 mg/m^3 for the concentrations of pyrethroid that could be detected without interference from organophosphorus or organochlorine insecticides. An alternative and more conventional approach would be to use a pumped device consisting of a filter (to trap droplets or particulates) in series with a packed tube (to trap vapour).

The use of a vacuum probe was described by Bengstone et al. (1983) to subsample pyrethroid-treated grain from several points within a silo for combination to give a composite sample. However, care is needed to obtain a representative sample using this procedure (GIFAP, 1981).

2.3.2 Sample storage

Storage stability experiments using untreated samples fortified with cyhalothrin (at 1.0 mg/kg) have shown that apples, cabbage, soil, and products of animal origin can be stored deep frozen at temperatures of -20 °C for periods of up to one year without residue loss (Sapiets, 1984a)

Particular problems in the handling of water samples have already been indicated and samples should be extracted and analysed as soon after sampling as possible.

2.4 Sample preparation

Forbes & Dutton (1985) reported details of the procedures used to process crop and soil samples, which have been treated with pyrethroid insecticides, for subsampling before extraction. Crops of high water content, e.g., fruit and vegetables, were chopped, dried, or puréed. Grain and oil seed crops (cotton seed and linseed) were frozen and ground to a powder, while crops of low water content, e.g., straw and tobacco, were finely divided in a rotary knife mill. Soil samples were mixed thoroughly and stones and plant debris removed. In all cases, care was taken to avoid localized overheating of the sample during processing. Sapiets et al. (1984) used a similar processing procedure for high water content crops and also applied this to meat and eggs. However, they draw attention to the importance of processing materials with high water content while still frozen to prevent separation of juice, which leads to sample inhomogeneity. Milk was thoroughly mixed before subsampling. In the limited number of other studies where details for preparation of pyrethroid-treated samples have been given, none of the procedures differ markedly from those described above. All of the procedures are equally applicable to cyhalothrin and lambda-cyhalothrin.

2.5 Gas chromatographic procedures for the determination of cyhalothrin residues

Details of GC procedures are described in the following subsections (Sapiets, 1984b,c, 1985a,b, 1986a,b).

2.5.1 Extraction

Representative subsamples of prepared crops or meat are blended for 2-5 min with a mixture of acetone and hexane (1 + 1 by volume). Dry materials are dampened with water. Soil is similarly extracted by refluxing with acetonitrile for 1 h. Extracts are then gravity filtered and partitioned with 5% sodium chloride solution to remove the acetone. The hexane extract is dried over anhydrous sodium sulfate.

Eggs are extracted by homogenizing for 5 min with acetonitrile. An aliquot is evaporated to dryness and redissolved in hexane.

Milk is extracted by homogenizing for 2 min in acetone and hexane (1:1 by volume). The solvent is dried over anhydrous sodium sulfate.

2.5.2 Clean-up

Column absorption chromatography on Florisil is used for cleaning up extracts from crops and soils, and cyhalothrin residues are eluted with a mixture of diethyl ether in hexane.

Extracts from crops with high lipid content, animal products, and difficult matrices, e.g., tobacco and hops, require preliminary clean-up by liquid-liquid partition procedures.

2.5.3 Determination

Residues of cyhalothrin in cleaned-up extracts are determined by GC/ECD using packed or capillary columns.

A variety of liquid phases have been found suitable for use with packed columns; these include OV-25, OV-101, OV-210, and OV-202. These are generally used at low loadings (3-5%) in the temperature range 230-250 °C, and retention times for cyhalothrin are normally less than 10 min. Glass columns should be used. On these packed columns cyhalothrin is eluted as a single peak.

Capillary columns will separate the two pairs of diastereoisomers (enantiomer pairs) of cyhalothrin to give two peaks. Lambda-cyhalothrin under the same conditions gives a single peak. Fused silica columns, 25 m long, coated with OV-101 have been found suitable when separate determination of diastereoisomers in the cyhalothrin residue is required. Retention times normally fall within the range of 10 to 30 min.

2.5.4 Limit of determination

The limit of determination of the methods for cyhalothrin residues in crops and animal products is set at

0.01 mg/kg on the basis of recovery experiments at low fortification levels (0.005-0.02 mg/kg) and background noise in the chromatograms. The limit of determination for soils is set at 0.005 to 0.01 mg/kg and for water is 10 ng/litre (ppt).

2.5.5 *Recoveries and interference*

The internal standardization procedure used in these methods determines the concentration of cyhalothrin or lambda-cyhalothrin relative to that of a known concentration of internal standard added to the sample prior to extraction. Correction for percentage recovery is thereby inherent for each individual sample. The repeatability of the procedure for most substrates is 2 to 3%. The methods have been found to be applicable to the determination of cyhalothrin in a wide variety of substrates without interference from endogenous natural products in the GC determination.

2.5.6 *Confirmation of residue identity*

Qualitative and quantitative confirmation of residue identity may be achieved by combined GC-MS operated in the selected ion monitoring mode.

3. SOURCES AND LEVELS OF HUMAN AND ENVIRONMENTAL EXPOSURE

3.1 Production levels and processes

No data on industrial production are available.

3.2 Uses

Cyhalothrin is a pyrethroid insecticide with a high level of activity (application rate up to 20 g/ha) against a wide range of *Lepidoptera, Hemiptera, Diptera*, and *Coleoptera* species. It also has some miticidal activity. Lambda-cyhalothrin has the same spectrum of insecticidal activity as cyhalothrin but it is more active. The compound is a stomach, contact, and residual insecticide. It shows adulticidal, ovicidal and, particularly, larvicidal activity.

Like other photostable synthetic pyrethroids, cyhalothrin and lambda-cyhalothrin are relatively stable to degradation in sunlight. This permits their use as practical tools in agriculture. The compound is not plant-systemic and has very little fumigant or translaminar activity.

Owing, in part, to its short persistence in soil and lack of systemic effect, the compound is of only limited value when used as a soil insecticide. It can, however, give useful control of cutworms when applied as a crop/ground spray. It has no molluscicidal or nematocidal activity.

Preventive treatments are generally more effective than curative treatments against major pests such as boring caterpillars or leaf miners. A programme of sprays is usually required, particularly during the more active growth stages of the plant and when the potential for re-infestation remains high.

Cyhalothrin has also found uses in public and animal health applications where it effectively controls a broad spectrum of insects, including cockroaches, flies, mosquitos, and ticks. It has high activity as a residual spray on inert surfaces.

3.3 Residues in food

Supervised trials have been carried out on a wide variety of crops, and comprehensive summaries of residue analysis in these trials can be found in the evaluation reports of the Joint FAO/WHO Meeting on Pesticide Residues (JMPR) (FAO/WHO 1985, 1986a).

Data reviewed by the JMPR showed that in studies on apples and on pears, when different rates of application were used in the same trial, initial residues reflected the different rates applied. When the spray programme was doubled from three to six applications per season, there was no increase in the lambda-cyhalothrin residue levels over those obtained with the three applications programme at the same rates. Lambda-cyhalothrin residue levels on apples often declined relatively slowly, although this was not always the case. There were no obvious differences in residue levels arising from the use of the different strengths of emulsion concentrate formulations or from the use of either low volume or high volume rates of application (FAO/WHO, 1986a,b).

3.4 Levels in the environment

3.4.1 *Air*

No specific data on air concentrations are available. Since cyhalothrin and lambda-cyhalothrin are of low vapour pressure, atmospheric levels of their vapour will be negligible.

3.4.2 *Water*

No specific data on water levels are available. Since cyhalothrin and lambda-cyhalothrin are insoluble in water and not mobile in soil, they are very unlikely to reach ground water.

3.4.3 *Soil*

No information on concentrations in soil is available.

4. ENVIRONMENTAL TRANSPORT, DISTRIBUTION, AND TRANSFORMATION

4.1 Transportation and distribution between media

The very low vapour pressure of cyhalothrin means that this compound will not enter the atmosphere.

Studies have shown that cyhalothrin and its soil degradation products do not leach through soils. ^{14}C-cyclopropane-labelled cyhalothrin was aerobically incubated for 30 days with a sandy loam (4.2% organic matter) and a loamy sand (2.0% organic matter). The incubated soils (rates equivalent to 0.04 and 0.05 kg cyhalothrin equivalents per ha for the sandy loam and loamy sand, respectively) were then applied to soil columns (30 cm long) and leached during a period of 9 weeks with 66 cm "rain". The radioactive residues more than 5 cm beneath the surface were below the limit of determination (i.e. < 0.47 ng cyhalothrin equivalents per g) in all the soil columns. Radioactive residues in the leachate samples were also generally below the limit of determination (i.e. < 0.023 ng cyhalothrin equivalent per ml) and represented less than 0.3% of the applied radiocarbon. Thus, cyhalothrin, lambda-cyhalothrin, and their degradation products have very low mobility in soil. On the basis of these data it is concluded that the agricultural use of cyhalothrin or lambda-cyhalothrin will not result in the leaching of either the parent compounds or their degradation products into ground water (Stevens & Bewick, 1985). Furthermore, if soils containing cyhalothrin are flooded, there is no release of cyhalothrin into the water (Hamer & Hill, 1985). Thus, residues of cyhalothrin in soil resulting from agricultural use will not be transported into other compartments of the environment.

4.2 Abiotic degradation

4.2.1 Hydrolysis and photodegradation in water

In studies by Collis & Leahey (1984), aqueous solutions of ^{14}C-cyclopropyl-labelled lambda-cyhalothrin, buffered at pH 5, 7, and 9, were maintained in the dark at 25° C for periods of up to 30 days. Acetonitrile (1%) was used as a co-solvent to facilitate dissolution in the water. Hydrolysis of lambda-cyhalothrin occurred rapidly in the pH 9 aqueous buffer solution (half-life, approximately 7 days) via ester cleavage of the molecule to yield (1*RS*)-*cis*-3-(*Z*-2-chloro-3,3,3-trifluoroprop-1-enyl)-2,2-dimethylcyclopropanecarboxylic acid. Rapid isomerization of the optical centre at the α-CN position also occurred at pH 9. At pH 7 no hydrolysis was detected, but slow isomerization did occur. At pH 5 no hydrolysis or isomerization was observed (Collis & Leahey, 1984).

When quartz flasks containing ^{14}C-cyclopropyl-labelled lambda-cyhalothrin in pH 5 buffer were exposed to sunlight for 30 days, the compound underwent photodegradation with a half-life of approximately 30 days. (1*RS*)-*cis*- and (1*RS*)-*trans*-3-(*ZE*-2-chloro-3,3,3-trifluoroprop-1-enyl)-2,2-dimethylcyclopropanecarboxylic acids and (*RS*)-α-amido-3-phenoxybenzyl (1*RS*)-*cis,trans*-3-(*ZE*-2-chloro-3,3,3-trifluoroprop-1-enyl)-2,2-dimethylcyclopropanecarboxylate were the major degradation products formed. Optical and geometrical isomerization of lambda-cyhalothrin occurred in the irradiated flasks. No photodegradation or photoisomerization was observed in a dark control flask (Curl et al., 1984a).

In studies by Hall & Leahey (1983), ^{14}C-cyhalothrin was incubated with two river water/sediment mixtures contained in quartz flasks. The flasks were either exposed to sunlight or were maintained under dark conditions by covering them with aluminium foil. In the dark, degradation of cyhalothrin was slow (over 80% remained unchanged after 32 days). However, when exposed to sunlight the cyhalothrin degraded with a half-life of approximately 20 days in both river water/sediment mixtures. The rate at which the parent compound was lost from the aqueous phase was, however, much faster than its rate of degradation in the whole water/sediment system. This was due to the ready absorption of cyhalothrin onto the sediment. The major degradation process was simple ester cleavage of the molecule, producing (1*RS*)-*cis*- and (1*RS*)-*trans*-3-(*ZE*-2-chloro-3,3,3-trifluoroprop-1-enyl)-2,2-dimethylcyclopropanecarboxylic acids. After 32 days of irradiation, these compounds together represented 36-47% of the radioactivity applied to the water/sediment systems. Some photoisomerization also occurred.

4.2.2 Photodegradation in soil

When thin-layer soil plates were treated with ^{14}C-cyclopropyl-labelled lambda-cyhalothrin and irradiated in a xenon arc apparatus or in sunlight, the half-life of lambda-cyhalothrin was less than 2 days in the xenon arc apparatus and less than 30 days in sunlight. (1*RS*)-*cis*-3-(*ZE*-2-chloro-3,3,3-trifluoroprop-1-enyl)-2,2-dimethylcyclopropane-carboxylic acid and (*RS*)-α-amido-3-phenoxybenzyl (1*RS*)-*cis*, *trans*-3-(*ZE*-2-chloro-3,3,3-trifluoroprop-1-enyl)-2,2-dimethylcyclopropanecarboxylate were the major degradation products (Curl et al., 1984b).

4.3 Biodegradation in soil

Cyhalothrin degradation in the outdoor environment may occur by either biological or photochemical processes. In most cases, biological processes are by far the most important, although photochemical reactions can sometimes contribute to the degradation of residues on exposed surfaces.

4.3.1 Degradation rate

At residue levels that are likely to occur under normal field conditions, cyhalothrin is degraded rapidly in soil. When a sandy loam soil was treated with ^{14}C-cyclopropyl-labelled cyhalothrin, only 28% of the recovered radioactivity was present as cyhalothrin after five weeks of incubation under aerobic conditions; 30% was evolved as ^{14}C-labelled carbon dioxide and 3.5% of the recovered radioactivity was due to 1*RS*-*cis*-3-(*Z*-2-chloro-3,3,3-trifluoroprop-1-enyl)-2,2-dimethylcyclopropanecarboxylic acid. Approximately 19% of the radioactivity was not extracted using acetonitrile at room temperature followed by soxhlet extraction with aqueous acetonitrile (Bewick & Zinner, 1981).

In a more recent and detailed study, ^{14}C-cyclopropyl-labelled cyhalothrin was applied to two soils (a sandy loam and a loamy sand) at 100 g/ha and incubated under both aerobic and flooded conditions at 20 °C. The sandy loam soil was also treated with cyhalothrin at 500 g/ha and, in a later experiment, treated separately with the two enantiomer pairs of cyhalothrin (one of which constitutes lambda-cyhalothrin). This soil was also incubated at 10 °C. All the isomers of cyhalothrin, including those that constitute lambda-cyhalothrin, were readily degraded in soil under a range of conditions. Half-lives for cyhalothrin at 20 °C in the sandy loam and loamy sand soils were 22 and 82 days, respectively. Degradation was somewhat slower in the sandy loam at higher rates (half-life: 42 days), lower temperature (half-life: 56 days) and under flooded conditions (half-life: 74 days). Lambda-cyhalothrin was degraded at about 70% the rate of the other enantiomer pair of cyhalothrin in the aerobic soils but at approximately the same rate under flooded conditions. In the aerobic soils, the principle degradative reactions were hydroxylation, yielding up to 11% of the applied radiocarbon as (*RS*)-α-cyano-3-(4-hydroxyphenoxy) benzyl *cis*-3-(*Z*-2-chloro-3,3,3-trifluoroprop-1-enyl)-2,2-dimethylcyclopropanecarboxylate (compound XV), and hydrolysis, yielding up to 7% as (*RS*)-*cis*-3-(Z-2-chloro-3,3,3-trifluoroprop-1-enyl)-2,2-dimethylcyclopropanecarboxylic acid (compound Ia). In the flooded soil, hydrolysis was the main degradative reaction (up to 18% of compound Ia in the soil phase), and hydroxylation was less important (only up to 1.4% of compound XV). Compound Ia was the only compound detected (up to 17%) in the aqueous phase of the flooded soils. No isomerization of the parent esters or their hydrolysis product was detected. The initial degradation products of cyhalothrin and lambda-cyhalothrin in the aerobic soils were rapidly further degraded with extensive mineralization (up to 70% in 26 weeks) to $^{14}CO_2$ (Bharti et al., 1985). Thus the acid moiety of cyhalothrin is readily mineralized in soil. The alcohol moiety of this compound is identical to that of cypermethrin. Studies with cypermethrin show that, after ester cleavage, the alcohol moiety released is readily mineralized to $^{14}CO_2$ (FAO/WHO, 1986a).

In a further study, when ^{14}C-cyclopropyl-labelled cyhalothrin was applied (at 100 g/ha) to a Japanese upland soil (a volcanic ash) and incubated under aerobic conditions at 20 °C, the half-life of cyhalothrin was approximately 100 days. The principle degradative reactions were hydroxylation, yielding up to 7% of the applied radiocarbon as compound XV, and hydrolysis, yielding up to ≈ 2% as compound Ia. The initial degradation products of cyhalothrin were further degraded with mineralization (up to 17% in 26 weeks) to $^{14}CO_2$ (Bharti & Bewick, 1986).

Four sites in the USA were treated with lambda-cyhalothrin (1.1 kg/ha), and soil was sampled and analysed at intervals up to 9 months after treatment. Residues remained in the top 15 cm of soil, except at one site where low residues immediately after treatment and at 2 days were attributed to contamination during sampling. Initial soil residues of 0.18 to 0.31 mg/kg declined to extremely low levels (< 0.01 to 0.02 mg/kg) during the course of the study, and at one site the residues were less than the limit of determination after 91 days (Fitzpatrick, 1985).

4.3.2 Degradation pathways

Degradation pathways for cyhalothrin and lambda-cyhalothrin in soil are shown in Figure 2.

4.4 Metabolism in plants

In studies by Leahey & French (1986a), soya bean plants were treated with ^{14}C-cyclopropane-labelled and ^{14}C-benzyl-labelled lambda-cyhalothrin. Two applications (18 days apart) were made by spraying an EC formulation at a rate of 20 g/ha. The plants were analysed at maturity, 39 days after the second application, when radioactive residues on the leaves ranged from 1.2 mg/kg (benzyl-labelled treatment) to 1.5 mg/kg (cyclopropane-labelled treatment). Very little radioactivity translocated into seeds (< 0.01 mg/kg).

In a similar experiment, in which cotton plants were treated with ^{14}C-cyclopropane-labelled and ^{14}C-benzyl-labelled lambda-cyhalothrin, three applications at a rate of 66 g/ha were made (at flowering and 3 and 7 weeks after flowering). The plants were analysed, at maturity, 30 days after the final application. The radioactive residues on the leaves at harvest were 3.7 mg/kg for the benzyl-labelled treatment and 4.1 mg/kg for the cyclopropane-

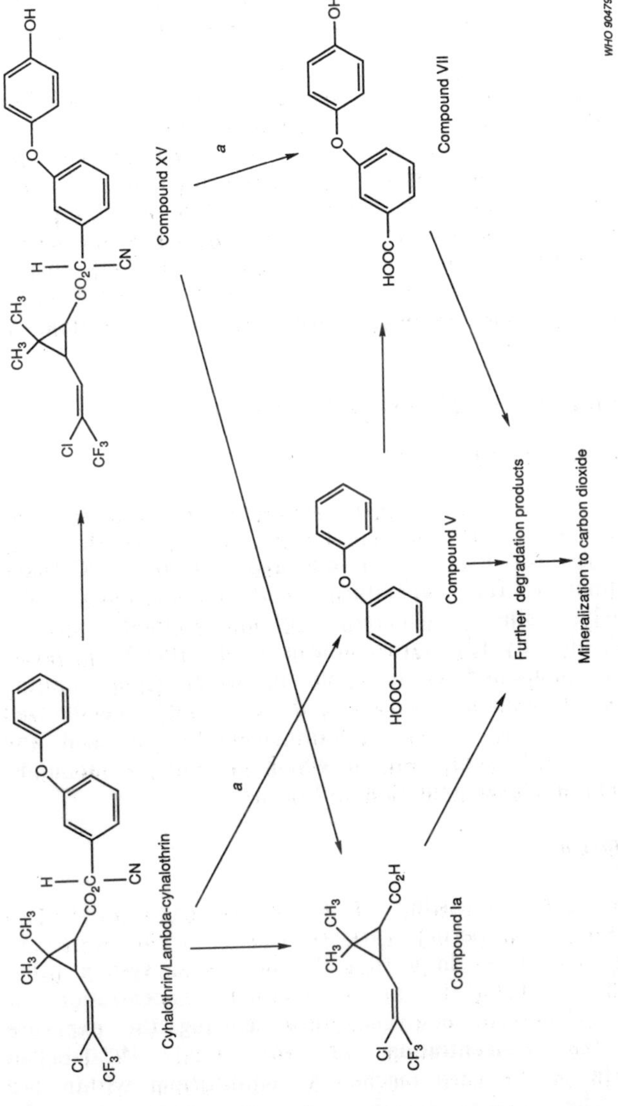

[a] presumably formed via cyanohydrin and aldehyde intermediates

Fig. 2. Proposed degradation pathways for cyhalothrin and lambda-cyhalothrin in soil.

labelled treatment. Very little radioactivity (< 0.03 mg/kg) was detected in the cotton seeds (Leahey & French, 1986b,c).

At harvest, the major constituents of the radioactive residue on the leaves of both cotton and soya bean were lambda-cyhalothrin and other isomeric forms of lambda-cyhalothrin resulting from photochemically initiated interconversions (soya: 52% benzyl-label, 45% cyclopropane-label; cotton: 52% benzyl-label, 37% cyclopropane-label). The metabolites detected on the leaves of both plants resulted from a range of hydrolytic and oxidative reactions. A metabolic pathway illustrating these reactions is shown in Fig. 3.

4.5 Bioaccumulation and biomagnification

4.5.1 *n-Octanol-water partition coefficient*

In common with other synthetic pyrethroids, the *n*-octanol-water partition coefficient of cyhalothrin is high; values for log P_{ow} of 6.9 and 7.0 at 20 °C have been obtained for cyhalothrin and lambda-cyhalothrin, respectively, using a generator column method (personal communication by ICI Agrochemicals to the IPCS). However, since the compound is insoluble in water (thus limiting exposures of aquatic species) and is rapidly metabolized in animal systems to the cyclopropanecarboxylic acid and 3-phenoxybenzoic acid, both of which are polar compounds, no problem of bioaccumulation will occur.

4.5.2 *Bioaccumulation*

In a study consisting of a 28-day exposure and a 28-day depuration period, carp *(Cyprinus carpio)* were exposed to cyhalothrin in a flow-through water system using ^{14}C-labelled cyhalothrin at a nominal concentration of 0.02 μg cyhalothrin equivalent/litre. During the exposure period, the concentration of the total ^{14}C-labelled cyhalothrin in the carp reached an equilibrium within 1-2 weeks. The bioconcentration factors measured were: 4250-7340 in the viscera, 490-850 in the muscle, 1020-2290 in the remainder of the body, and 1660-2240 in the whole fish. Rapid depuration of residues was observed; the biological half-life of the total ^{14}C-labelled cyhalothrin

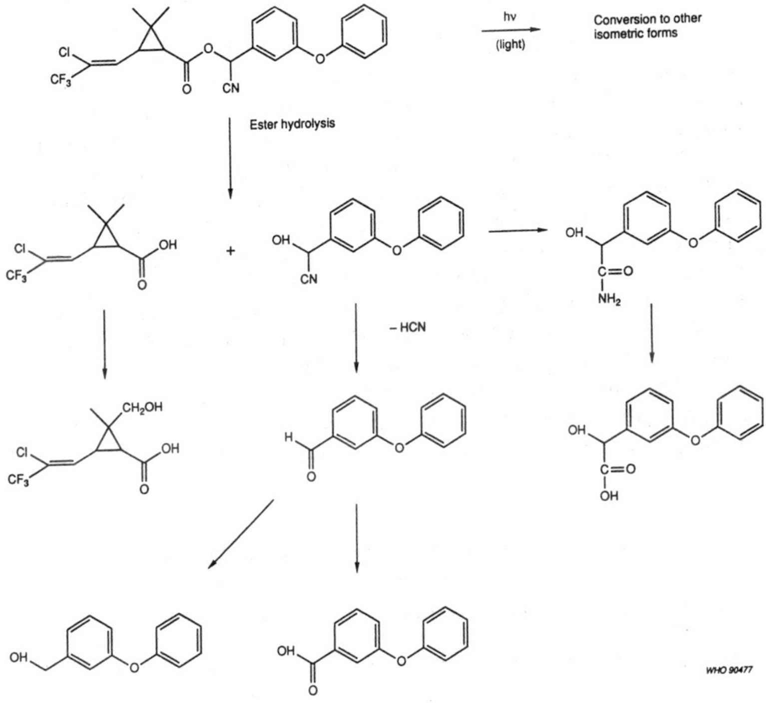

Fig. 3. Metabolism of cyhalothrin in plants.

was 9 days in the viscera, muscle, and whole fish (Yamauchi et al., 1984a).

The accumulation of cyhalothrin and its degradation products in channel catfish and *Daphnia magna* has been investigated in a soil-water system. ^{14}C-cyclopropane-labelled cyhalothrin was applied at 50 g ai per ha and aerobically incubated in soil for 3 weeks prior to flooding. Channel catfish and *Daphnia magna* were introduced for exposure periods of 31 and 28 days, respectively, after which the fish and daphnids were transferred to an uncontaminated system for depuration periods of 42 and 7 days, respectively. Soil, water, fish, and daphnids were analysed for ^{14}C-residues. Prior to flooding, ^{14}C-labelled residues in soil decreased to 60-70% of that applied, 40% of which remained as extractable cyhalothrin. Following flooding of the soil, ^{14}C-labelled residues in the water increased throughout the exposure period, reaching a level of 8% of the applied radioactivity. No parent cyhalothrin was detected in the water; the only product comprising more than 1% of the applied radioactivity was *cis*-3-(*ZE*-2-chloro-3,3,3-trifluoroprop-1-enyl-2,2-dimethylcyclopropanecarboxylic acid, which represented up to 5.3% of the applied radioactivity. During exposure, the maximum bioconcentration factors in whole fish and daphnids were 19 and 194, respectively (Table 2). The concentration of ^{14}C-residues in fish and daphnids decreased during the depuration period, the half-lives being approximately 7 days and 1 day, respectively (Table 3) (Hamer & Hill, 1985).

Table 2. Bioconcentration factors for cyhalothrin in *Daphnia* and fish

Exposure phase (days)	*Daphnia*	Fish muscle	Fish viscera	Whole fish
1	93	2	20	17
3	194	3	28	7
7	158	6	45	10
14	62	7	66	19
21	47	5	28	10
28	29	7	49	8
31	NR	7	48	9

From: Hamer & Hill (1985)
NR = not recorded.

Table 3. Concentration of ^{14}C-residues in *Daphnia* and fish tissues

Depuration phase (days)	% of tissue level on final day of exposure			
	Daphnia	Fish muscle	Fish viscera	Whole fish
1	56	105	60	80
3	29	66	53	64
4	NR	NR	NR	61
7	11	51	4	38
14	NR	32	4	37
21	NR	31	6	27
42	NR	20	2	14

From: Hamer & Hill (1985)
NR = not recorded.

5. KINETICS AND METABOLISM

5.1 Absorption, distribution, and excretion

5.1.1 Rat

In studies by Harrison (1981, 1984a,b), groups of six male and six female Alderley Park rats received a single oral dose (1 or 25 mg/kg) of radiolabelled cyhalothrin in corn oil. As it was known that the metabolism of related pyrethroids involves extensive cleavage of the ester bond, duplicate experiments were performed using two forms of cyhalothrin labelled with ^{14}C in the acid (^{14}C-cyclopropyl) or alcohol (^{14}C-benzyl) portions of the ester. Excreta (urine, faeces and, in selected animals, expired air) were collected for up to 7 days after dosing and analysed for total radioactivity and metabolites by liquid scintillation counting and thin-layer chromatography. Blood samples were also collected at various times up to 48 h and analysed for total radioactivity and unchanged cyhalothrin.

Following oral administration of cyhalothrin, absorption was variable but accounted for about 55% of the dose. The proportions absorbed were similar at both dose levels.

Excretion was rapid for both ^{14}C-cyclopropyl- and ^{14}C-benzyl-labelled cyhalothrin at both dose levels, although excretion rates were faster with the ^{14}C-benzyl label than with the ^{14}C-cyclopropyl label. Urinary excretion accounted for approximately 20-40% of the dose and faecal excretion for 40-65% of the dose during the first 7 days. Peak blood concentrations of radioactivity were reached within 4-7 h, and by 48 h these concentrations had declined to 10% or less of peak values. A small proportion of an oral dose (2-3%) was retained in the animals after seven days; analysis of twelve different tissues indicated that this radioactivity was present mainly in white fat.

Results from a study in which rats were dosed subcutaneously indicated that some of the dose was excreted via the bile.

In a further experiment to study the excretion and tissue accumulation of cyhalothrin (1 mg/kg per day by gavage), groups of six male and six female rats received daily doses of ^{14}C-benzyl-labelled or ^{14}C-cyclopropyl-labelled cyhalothrin for 14 days. Urine and faecal samples were collected every 24 h up to 7 days after the final dose. Groups of animals were killed 2, 5, and 7 days after the final dose and a range of tissues were removed for measurement of residual radioactivity. Fat samples were analysed by HPLC for unchanged cyhalothrin. The results demonstrated that the excretion of ^{14}C-material after multiple oral dosing was similar to that which followed a single dose. Slightly higher overall excretion in urine (up to 50% of the administered dose) was probably due to more consistent oral absorption in this study. A large proportion of the oral dose of cyhalothrin was rapidly eliminated from the body. Analysis of tissue residues revealed that the small proportion (< 5%) of the dose retained in white fat was unchanged cyhalothrin, which was eliminated from this tissue with a half-life of about 23 days (Harrison, 1981, 1984a,b).

A further study was undertaken in the rat to explore the retention, in fat, of cyhalothrin and lambda-cyhalothrin. Groups of male rats received daily oral doses of ^{14}C-cyclopropyl-labelled cyhalothrin (1 mg/kg per day) for up to 119 days. At intervals during and after the dosing period, groups of three rats were killed and the concentrations of radioactivity in the liver, kidney, fat, and blood were determined. Additionally the concentration in fat of lambda-cyhalothrin and its opposite enantiomer pair (enantiomer pair A) was measured by high-pressure liquid chromatography. Levels of radioactivity in the blood remained fairly constant and low (approximately 0.2 µg cyhalothrin equivalents per g) throughout the dosing period. In the liver and kidney, the radioactivity reached a plateau, after approximately 70 days, at a level corresponding to approximately 2.5 µg cyhalothrin equivalents per g liver and 1.2 µg per g kidney. The concentration of cyhalothrin in fat at the end of the dosing period was approximately 10 µg/g. After the cessation of dosing, levels of radioactivity in the liver, kidney, and blood declined rapidly. In fat, the levels declined more slowly with an elimination half-life of 30 days. The radioactive material in fat was unchanged cyhalothrin; the ratio of enantiomeric pairs, one of which was lambda-cyhalothrin, was not significantly different from that in the dosing solution, indicating that the rate of metabolism of lambda-cyhalothrin was the same as cyhalothrin and that there was no preferential accumulation of lambda-cyhalothrin (Prout, 1984).

A comparison of the absorption, distribution, excretion, and metabolism of lambda-cyhalothrin and cyhalothrin was made to establish whether the single enantiomer pair lambda-cyhalothrin differed from cyhalothrin (a 50:50 mixture of lambda-cyhalothrin and the opposite enantiomer pair A) (Prout & Howard, 1985). One group of four male rats was given a single oral dose of ^{14}C-cyclopropyl-labelled lambda-cyhalothrin (1 mg/kg); a second group of four male rats was given ^{14}C-cyclopropyl-labelled lambda-cyhalothrin (1 mg/kg) plus the unlabelled enantiomeric pair A (1 mg/kg); and a third group of four male rats was given a single oral dose of a 50:50 mixture of ^{14}C-cyclopropyl-labelled lambda-cyhalothrin and ^{14}C-labelled enantiomeric pair A (i.e. ^{14}C-cyclopropyl-labelled cyhalothrin at 1 mg/kg). The urinary and faecal excretion of radioactivity was monitored in all three groups for three days and the residual radioactivity was then determined in selected tissues. The metabolite profile of the excreta was determined by thin-layer chromatography. The results of this study indicate that co-administration of enantiomer pair A with lambda-cyhalothrin had little or no effect upon the absorption, distribution, or tissue retention of radioactivity, and there was no effect upon the metabolite profile of lambda-cyhalothrin. Similarly, the absorption, distribution, excretion, and metabolism of cyhalothrin was indistinguishable from that of lambda-cyhalothrin, thus confirming the results of the bioaccumulation study of Prout (1984).

5.1.2 Dog

The absorption, distribution, excretion, and metabolism of cyhalothrin have been studied in the dog. As in the rat studies, the experiments were duplicated using cyhalothrin labelled either in the acid (^{14}C-cyclopropyl) or alcohol (^{14}C-benzyl) moieties of the molecule.

Groups of three male and three female beagle dogs were given a single oral dose of cyhalothrin (1 mg/kg or 10 mg/kg) and, after a 3-week interval, a further single intravenous administration of 0.1 mg/kg. Samples of blood and excreta were collected for 7 days after dosing and were analysed for total radioactivity. The proportions of unchanged cyhalothrin and of metabolites in urine and faeces were determined by thin-layer chromatography. The identity of major metabolites was confirmed by mass spectrometry.

The absorption of cyhalothrin after oral administration was variable. The degree of absorption was difficult to assess but was within the range 48%-80%. Excretion of radioactivity after both oral and intravenous dosing was initially rapid, with most of the administered radioactivity being excreted in the first 48 h after dosing. After 7 days, a mean of 82-93% had been excreted (Harrison, 1984c).

5.1.3 Cow

After twice daily oral ingestion of ^{14}C-benzyl- or ^{14}C-cyclopropyl-labelled cyhalothrin (1 mg/kg per day for 7 days), absorption of the insecticide by cows was apparently slow and incomplete. Approximately 50% of the dosed radioactivity was excreted in the faeces, mainly as unchanged cyhalothrin, but only small amounts were detected in the bile. With both labelled forms, most of the radioactive material was rapidly eliminated in the urine (27%) and faeces (49%) within 24 h of each daily dose. Only a very small proportion of the dose was secreted in the milk (0.8%) and this was found to be unchanged cyhalothrin. Tissue residues of radioactive material were low and were in the following order: fats > liver > kidney > blood > muscle. Residues in fat consisted of unchanged cyhalothrin. The liver and kidney contained small amounts of cyhalothrin, but the residues were largely due to a number of ester-cleavage metabolites that were probably present because the animals were still actively metabolizing and eliminating a significant fraction of the most recent day's intake of cyhalothrin. The almost two-fold difference in the plasma levels of total radiolabelled components obtained with the different labelled forms suggests that little cyhalothrin was present in blood. The ester link must therefore be hydrolysed very rapidly, apart from a small fraction that is distributed into fatty tissues (Harrison, 1984d).

In studies by Sapiets (1985c), Friesian cows were fed for up to thirty consecutive days on diets containing lambda-cyhalothrin at 1, 5, and 25 mg/kg. Lambda-cyhalothrin residues in milk correlated well with dietary inclusion rates, the mean plateau residue levels being 0.02 mg/kg, 0.09 mg/kg, and 0.52 mg/kg, respectively, for the three dietary inclusion rates. Lambda-cyhalothrin residue levels in milk did not accumulate, and they declined when feeding of the treated diet ceased. At the end of the 30 days, three cows from each group were sacrificed. The remaining two cows from the high-dose group were fed an untreated diet for a further 14 days before they too were slaughtered. Lambda-cyhalothrin residue levels in the tissues of the sacrificed animals were as shown in Table 4.

5.2 Metabolism

The metabolic pathways that have been established for cyhalothrin in mammals are summarized in Fig. 4.

5.2.1 Rat

Identification of the metabolites produced in the rat studies of Harrison (described in section 5.1.1) revealed that, following oral administration, unabsorbed cyhalothrin was eliminated unchanged via the faeces. The absorbed material was rapidly and extensively metabolized and no unchanged cyhalothrin was present in urine or bile. The main route of metabolism was, as anticipated, via hydrolysis of the ester linkage (Fig. 4). The cyclopropanecarboxylic acid moiety was subsequently excreted via the urine as the glucuronide conjugate. This material accounted for about 50% of the radioactivity in urine following dosing with ^{14}C-cyclopropyl-labelled cyhalothrin. The 3-phenoxybenzyl moiety was further metabolized by loss of the nitrile group, oxidation of the aldehyde formed to a carboxylic acid, aromatic hydroxylation at the 4′position, and formation of the 4-*O*-sulfate conjugate

Table 4. Lambda-cyhalothrin residues (mg/kg) in cow tissues[a]

Dietary feeding rate (mg/kg)	Abductor muscle	Pectoral muscle	Subcutaneous fat	Peritoneal fat	Liver	Kidney
1.0	< 0.01	< 0.01	0.01-0.21	0.07-0.50	< 0.01-0.03	0.01-0.02
5.0	0.01-0.03	0.03-0.07	0.44-0.81	0.95-1.8	< 0.01	0.01-0.07
25.0	0.08-0.14	0.02-0.41	1.3-4.6	3.9-7.9	0.06-0.10	0.09-0.43
25.0 + 14-day recovery period	< 0.01-0.05	< 0.01-0.03	0.03-1.1	0.47-2.6	< 0.01	0.10-0.20
Control	< 0.01	< 0.01	< 0.01-0.02	< 0.01-0.07	< 0.01	< 0.01

[a] From: Sapiets (1985c).

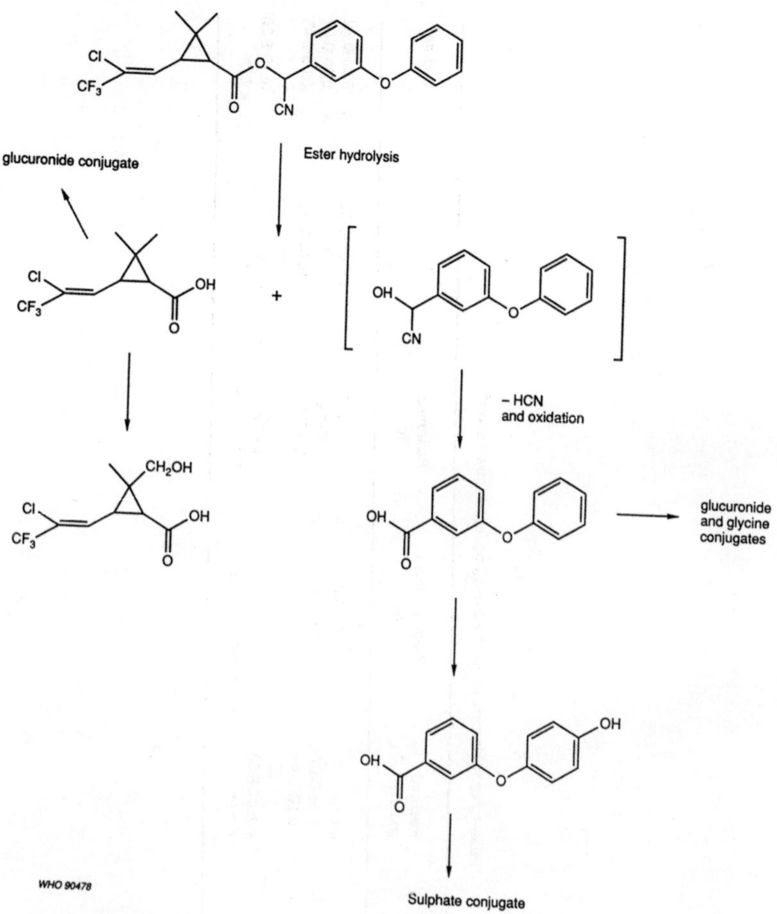
Cl
CF3
O
O
CN
Ester hydrolysis
glucuronide conjugate
OH
+
OH
CN
- HCN
and oxidation
CH2OH
glucuronide
and glycine
conjugates
Sulphate conjugate
WHO 90478

Fig. 4. Metabolism of cyhalothrin in mammals (postulated intermediate shown in square brackets).

of 3-(4-hydroxyphenoxy)benzoic acid. This conjugate accounted for approximately 75% of the urinary radioactivity following dosing with ^{14}C-benzyl-labelled cyhalothrin. No metabolite containing the ester function was detected (Harrison, 1983).

5.2.2 Dog

The main route of metabolism after oral administration is, as in the rat, via cleavage of the ester bond. After intravenous administration (0.1 mg/kg body weight), the patterns of metabolites in urine were very similar to those seen in the oral studies. Very little unchanged compound was present in the faeces or urine. The phenoxybenzyl moiety was further metabolized as in the rat; the main metabolites were *N*-(3-phenoxybenzyl) glycine, 3-(4-hydroxyphenoxy)benzoic acid and its sulfate conjugate, 3-phenoxybenzoyl glucuronide, and a little free 3-phenoxybenzoic acid. Other conjugated metabolites were also present. The cyclopropane acid moiety was extensively metabolized to produce 11 metabolites. These included the cyclopropane acid glucuronide and other conjugated metabolites. Thus, the metabolism of cyhalothrin is dominated by cleavage of the ester bond (Fig. 4). Subsequent metabolism of the products is similar both to that of other pyrethroids and to the fate of cyhalothrin in other species (Harrison, 1984c).

5.2.3 Cow

In common with other structurally related pyrethroids, the main routes of metabolism of cyhalothrin in the cow have been found to be similar to those observed in rats and dogs, i.e cleavage of the ester bond with subsequent excretion of the cyclopropyl carboxylic moiety, either free, hydroxylated, or as a glucuronide conjugate. The phenoxybenzyl moiety was further metabolized by loss of the nitrile group and excreted as free 3-phenoxybenzoic acid and its amino acid conjugates, or after aromatic hydroxylation probably at the 4′position. Cyhalothrin itself gives rise to residues in fats; this is consistent with the lipophilic properties of cyhalothrin compared to those of its more polar metabolites (Harrison, 1984d).

5.2.4 Goat

In a study by Leahey et al. (1985), a goat was dosed orally for seven days with ^{14}C-cyclopropyl-labelled lambda-cyhalothrin at a rate equivalent to approximately

11 mg/kg diet. During dosing, the maximum residue level in the milk was 0.27 mg cyhalothrin equivalents/kg (mean value during days 3-7: 0.21 mg/kg), virtually all of which was characterized as lambda-cyhalothrin. When the goat was slaughtered 16 h after receiving the final dose, residues in the tissues, expressed in cyhalothrin equivalents, were: meat, 0.024-0.028 mg/kg; fat, 0.13-0.44 mg/kg; liver, 0.34-0.35 mg/kg; kidney, 0.20 mg/kg. The residues in meat and fat were due mainly to lambda-cyhalothrin. However, in the liver and kidney, intact pyrethroid accounted for only a small part of the residue. (1*RS*)-*cis*-(*Z*-2-chloro-3,3,3-trifluoroprop-1-enyl)-2,2-dimethylcyclopropanecarboxylic acid and 3-(2-chloro-3,3,3-trifluoroprop-1-enyl)-2-hydroxymethyl-2-methylcyclopropanecarboxylic acid were the major components of the residue identified in liver and kidney.

5.2.5 Fish

In an accumulation study by Leahey & Parker (1985), carp were maintained in a flow-through water system containing ^{14}C-cyclopropyl-labelled cyhalothrin (at a level of 20 ng/g) for 28 days. Results showed that radioactive residues in muscle, head, and viscera were 0.035, 0.050, and 0.115 mg/kg, respectively. The major part of the ^{14}C-residue (50-65%) was characterized as cyhalothrin, a further 10-19% consisting of the compound Ia (Fig. 2).

6. EFFECTS ON ORGANISMS IN THE ENVIRONMENT

6.1 Aquatic organisms

6.1.1 Microorganisms

It has been shown that lambda-cyhalothrin, at a concentration of 1.0 mg/litre, does not affect the growth of the single-celled green alga *Selenastrum capricornutum* over a period of 96 h (Thompson & Williams, 1985).

6.1.2 Invertebrates

6.1.2.1 Acute toxicity

Aquatic invertebrates show a wide range of susceptibility to cyhalothrin and lambda-cyhalothrin. The data are summarized in Table 5.

6.1.2.2 Long-term toxicity

The effects of lambda-cyhalothrin on the survival, growth, and reproduction of *Daphnia magna* were investigated for a period of 21 days in a static water test with daily renewal of test solutions. The nominal concentrations tested were 0, 2.5, 5.0, 10.0, 20.0, and 40.0 ng/litre. Lambda-cyhalothrin affected all three parameters at a nominal concentration of 40 ng/litre, but no effects were noted at 2.5 ng/litre. Chemical analysis suggested that the daphnids were exposed to about 60% of the nominal concentration. These results show that the life-cycle no-observed-effect level of lambda-cyhalothrin for daphnids is of the order of 2.5 ng/litre (Hamer et al., 1985b).

6.1.3 Fish

6.1.3.1 Acute toxicity

Cyhalothrin and lambda-cyhalothrin are very toxic to fish in clean water under laboratory conditions. The available data, summarized in Table 6, demonstrate a similar high acute toxicity for both cold and warm water species of fish.

Table 5. Acute toxicity of cyhalothrin and lambda-cyhalothrin for aquatic invertebrates

Species	Stage	Temperature (°C)	Test substance	Test system	48-h LC_{50} (ng/litre)	Reference
Freshwater						
Water flea (*Daphnia pulex*)	< 24 h	20	cyhalothrin 5% WP	static	160	Yamauchi et al. (1984d)
Water flea (*Daphnia magna*)	12 h (± 12 h)	20	technical cyhalothrin	static	380	Williams & Thompson (1981)
Water flea (*Daphnia magna*)	< 24 h	20	technical lambda-cyhalothrin	static	360	Farrelly et al. (1984)
	< 24 h	20	lambda-cyhalothrin 5% EC	static	90[a]	Farrelly et al. (1985)
	< 24 h	20	lambda-cyhalothrin 13% EC	static	90[a]	Farrelly et al. (1985)
Freshwater shrimp (*Gammarus pulex*)	5 mm	15	^{14}C-lambda-cyhalothrin	flow-through	8	Hamer et al. (1985a)
Marine						
Mysid shrimp (*Mysidopsis bahia*)	< 48 h	25	^{14}C-lambda-cyhalothrin	flow-through	7.5	Thompson (1985)

[a] Concentration of active ingredient.

Table 6. Acute toxicity of cyhalothrin and lambda-cyhalothrin to fish

Species	Weight (g)	Test substance and vehicle	Temperature (°C)	96-h LC_{50} (µg/litre)	Reference
Rainbow trout (*Salmo gairdneri*)	0.32-1.37	technical cyhalothrin dispersed via acetone	12	0.54	Hill (1981a)
	0.30-1.48	technical lambda-cyhalothrin dispersed via acetone	12	0.24	Hill (1984a)
	0.99-2.32	lambda-cyhalothrin 2.5% EC dispersed in water	16	0.39	Hill (1985a)
	1.28-4.78	lambda-cyhalothrin 13% EC dispersed in water	12	0.44	Hill (1985b)
	0.87-4.09	lambda-cyhalothrin 5% EC dispersed in water	16	0.93	Hill (1985c)
Carp (*Cyprinus carpio*)	5.2	technical cyhalothrin dispersed via dimethylformamide	23-35	1.34[a]	Takeda Chemical Co. Ltd. (1979)
	5.4	cyhalothrin 5% WP	25	1.1	Yamauchi et al. (1984b)
	1.48-5.8	lambda-cyhalothrin 2.5% EC dispersed in water	22	0.54	Hill (1985d)
	3.92-7.28	lambda-cyhalothrin 5% EC dispersed in water	22	0.50	Hill (1985e)
Bluegill sunfish (*Lepomis macrochirus*)	0.23-0.84	technical cyhalothrin dispersed via acetone	22	0.46	Reynolds (1984)
	0.7-2.6	technical lambda-cyhalothrin dispersed via acetone	22	0.21	Hill (1984b)
	0.47-2.06	lambda-cyhalothrin 13% EC dispersed in water	22	0.28	Hill (1985f)
Sheephead minnow (*Cyprinodon variegatus*)	0.32-0.91	technical lambda-cyhalothrin dispersed via acetone	22	0.81	Hill (1985g)

[a] 72-h LC_{50}.

6.1.3.2 Long-term toxicity

Sheepshead minnow *Cyprinodon variegatus* embryos and larvae were continuously exposed (through 28 days post hatch) to mean measured lambda-cyhalothrin concentrations of 0.04, 0.07, 0.14, 0.25, and 0.38 μg/litre, in a flow-through system. The test was performed in duplicate. Assessments were made of percentage hatch and survival of embryos and of total length and weight of the larvae at the completion of the study. Hatchability was not affected ($P < 0.05$) at any concentration in the carrier dimethyl-formamide or dilution water controls, percentage hatch ranging from 81.3% to 100%. Larval survival was not significantly affected. A significant effect ($P < 0.05$) was found on the weight of the larvae at the highest concentration tested, but not at any other concentration. On the basis of these data the NOEL was 0.25 μg/litre and the lowest-observed-effect level (LOEL) was 0.38 μg/litre (Hill et al., 1985).

6.1.4 Model ecosystem

Cyhalothrin is readily adsorbed onto soil and suspended particles, which in consequence significantly reduces its toxicity to aquatic organisms (Yamauchi et al., 1984c). *Daphnia pulex* and *Cyprinus carpio* were used in four different systems to test this experimentally (Table 7). The median lethal concentrations (LC_{50}) were calculated, immobilization being used as the end-point for *Daphnia pulex*.

6.2 Terrestrial organisms

6.2.1 Birds

6.2.1.1 Acute toxicity

The toxicity of single oral doses of cyhalothrin and lambda-cyhalothrin for birds is summarized in Table 8.

The 5-day dietary LC_{50} for cyhalothrin and lambda-cyhalothrin has been measured in *Anas platyrhynchos* and *Colinus virginianus* (Table 9).

Table 7. Effect of soil on the toxicity (72-h LC_{50} in μg/litre) of cyhalothrin to *Daphnia pulex* and *Cyprinus carpio* [a]

Conditions	*Daphnia pulex*	*Cyprinus carpio*
Application to water surface (without soil)	0.4	9
Application to water surface (soil undisturbed)	1.0	32
Application to water surface (soil suspended)	16	57
Application to soil (soil undisturbed)	70	642

[a] From: Yamauchi et al (1984c).

Table 8. Oral toxicity of cyhalothrin and lambda-cyhalothrin for birds

Species	Age	Test substance and vehicle	Observation period	LD_{50} (mg/kg body weight)	References
Domestic hen (*Gallus domesticus*)	adult	cyhalothrin in corn oil	14 days	> 10 000	Roberts et al. (1982)
Mallard duck (*Anas platyrhynchos*)	adult	cyhalothrin in corn oil	14 days	> 5000	Roberts & Fairley (1981)
Mallard duck (*Anas platyrhynchos*)	adult	lambda-cyhalothrin in corn oil	14 days	> 3950	Roberts & Fairley (1984)

Table 9. Dietary LC_{50} of cyhalothrin and lambda-cyhalothrin for birds

Species	Age	Test substance	Observation period (post treatment)	LC_{50} (mg/kg diet)	Reference
Mallard duck (*Anas platyrhynchos*)	10 days	cyhalothrin	3 days	14 000	Roberts et al. (1981a)
Mallard duck (*Anas platyrhynchos*)	8 days	lambda-cyhalothrin	4 days	3948	Roberts et al. (1985a)
Bobwhite quail (*Colinus virginianus*)	10 days	cyhalothrin	3 days	> 7530	Roberts et al. (1981b)
Bobwhite quail (*Colinus virginianus*)	11 days	lambda-cyhalothrin	3 days	> 5300	Roberts et al. (1985b)

6.2.2 Honey-bees

Cyhalothrin and lambda-cyhalothrin have been shown to be toxic to honey-bees (*Apis mellifera*) in laboratory tests (Table 10).

Table 10. Toxicity of cyhalothrin and lambda-cyhalothrin for honey-bees (expressed as 24-h LD_{50} in μg ai per bee)

Formulation	Topical application	Oral administration	Reference
Technical cyhalothrin	0.027	-	Smart & Stevenson (1982)
Technical lambda-cyhalothrin	0.051	0.97	Gough et al. (1984)
Lambda-cyhalothrin EC (5%)	0.095	0.57	Gough et al. (1984)

In common with other pyrethroids, the high laboratory toxicity of lambda-cyhalothrin is not translated into a significant field hazard to bees. In two trials on flowering rape, lambda-cyhalothrin (JF 9509) EC was applied, at midday, by helicopter at a concentration of 10 g ai/ha to fields where hives of honey-bees were located. A toxic standard and untreated control were used for comparison. Bees were actively foraging during spraying, and the hives were oversprayed. Mortality, foraging activity, activity at the hive, and brood development were monitored before and after treatment, and pollen, honey, and wax were analyzed for residues. Apart from a suppression of foraging lasting up to 1.5 h, the lambda-cyhalothrin formulation had no effect on the bees, whereas the toxic standard killed large numbers. Only low levels of residues were detected (pollen, 0.44 μg/g; honey, 0.01 μg/g; wax, 0.01 μg/g). It was concluded that, at 10 g ai/ha, lambda-cyhalothrin formulation (JF 9509) EC is non-hazardous to honey-bees on flowering rape (Gough et al., 1985).

6.2.3 Earthworms

Three annual applications of lambda-cyhalothrin at rates of up to 250 g ai/ha to field plots had no adverse effect on populations of individual species of earthworms or total earthworm numbers or weight (Coulson et al., 1986).

6.2.4 *Higher plants*

No phytotoxic effects have been reported.

7. EFFECTS ON EXPERIMENTAL ANIMALS AND *IN VITRO* TEST SYSTEMS

7.1 Single exposures

7.1.1 Oral

The acute oral toxicity of cyhalothrin and lambda-cyhalothrin in corn oil has been determined for several species (Table 11). The toxicity of cyhalothrin is moderate (LD_{50} values: rat, 144-243 mg/kg; mouse, 37-62 mg/kg), whereas that of lambda-cyhalothrin is higher (LD_{50} values: rat, 56-79 mg/kg; mouse, 20 mg/kg). Signs of intoxication are characteristic of type II pyrethroid toxicity and included piloerection, subdued behaviour, ataxia, unsteady gait, salivation, incontinence, scouring, and chromodacryorrhoea.

Table 11. Acute oral toxicity of technical cyhalothrin and lambda-cyhalothrin in corn oil

Species	Test substance	LD_{50} (mg/kg body weight)	Reference
Rat	cyhalothrin	243 (male) 144 (female)	Nixon & Jackson (1981a)
Rat	lambda-cyhalothrin	79 (male) 56 (female)	Southwood (1985)
Mouse	cyhalothrin	36.7 (male) 62.3 (female)	Nixon & Jackson (1981a)
Mouse	lambda-cyhalothrin	19.9 (male) 19.9 (female)	Southwood (1984)
Guinea-pig	cyhalothrin	> 5000 (male)	Nixon & Jackson (1981a)
Rabbit	cyhalothrin	> 1000 (female)	Nixon & Jackson (1981a)

7.1.2 Percutaneous

The percutaneous toxicity of cyhalothrin and lambda-cyhalothrin is summarized in Table 12. Signs of intoxication were similar to those seen after oral ingestion,

Table 12. Percutaneous toxicity of technical cyhalothrin and lambda-cyhalothrin in polyethylene glycol paste

Species	Test substance	LD_{50} (mg/kg body weight)	Reference
Rat	cyhalothrin	1000-2000 (male) 200-2000 (female)	Nixon & Jackson (1981a)
Rat	lambda-cyhalothrin	632 (male) 696 (female)	Barber (1985)
Rabbit	cyhalothrin	> 2000 (male) > 2000 (female)	Nixon & Jackson (1981a)

and included incontinence, scouring, dehydration, subdued behaviour, curvature of the spine, unsteady gait, nervous appearance, piloerection, and increased vocalization when handled.

7.1.3 *Intraperitoneal*

The intraperitoneal LD_{50} of cyhalothrin to rats is in the range of 250 to 750 mg/kg. Responses of 0% or 100% mortality were observed at all but one dose, and so no precise value for the LD_{50} could be given. The highest dose with no mortality was 250 mg/kg and the lowest dose with 100% mortality was 750 mg/kg (Nixon & Jackson, 1981a).

7.2 Irritation and sensitization

7.2.1 *Irritation*

Undiluted technical cyhalothrin is a mild irritant to occluded rabbit skin (both intact and abraded) but is non-irritant to occluded rat skin (intact) (Jackson & Nixon, 1981). Technical cyhalothrin is a moderate irritant to the rabbit eye without irrigation and is a mild irritant when irrigated for one minute, 20 to 30 seconds after instillation of the material (Jackson, 1981).

Technical lambda-cyhalothrin is non-irritant to occluded rabbit skin without abrasion (Pritchard, 1985a). It is a mild irritant to the rabbit eye (Pritchard, 1985b).

7.2.2 Sensitization

A skin sensitization test with cyhalothrin on guinea-pigs, using the procedure of Buehler, indicated that cyhalothrin has skin-sensitizing potential (Nixon & Jackson, 1981b). In guinea-pigs that had been previously induced with undiluted cyhalothrin technical material, using the Magnusson and Kligman maximization test, a moderate sensitization response was elicited. When lambda-cyhalothrin was tested for skin sensitization on guinea-pigs, using the maximization procedure of Magnusson and Kligmann, it was shown to have no sensitization potential (Pritchard, 1984).

7.3 Short-term exposures

7.3.1 Oral

7.3.1.1 Rat

When groups of male and female rats were fed diets containing cyhalothrin at levels up to 750 mg/kg for 28 days, symptoms of toxicity shown by animals receiving doses of 250 mg/kg diet or more included high stepping gait, ataxia, and hypersensitivity to external stimuli. These effects were dose related and some mortality occurred at the highest dose level. The clinical signs were not accompanied by histopathological changes in the nervous system. Thymic atrophy, adrenal enlargement with vacuolization, and incomplete spermatogenesis occurred with the highest dose. An adaptive change was present in the liver as judged by an increase in liver weight, proliferation of smooth endoplasmic reticulum, and an increase in the activity of the xenobiotic-metabolizing enzyme, aminopyrine-*N*-demethylase (APDM). These effects occurred at doses of 100 mg/kg or more, and there was some evidence for this type of change at 20 mg/kg (Tinson et al., 1984).

When groups of 20 male and 20 female Wistar rats were fed cyhalothrin (89% pure) at dietary concentrations of 0, 10, 50, and 250 mg/kg for 90 days, only male rats fed 250 mg/kg showed significantly reduced body weight gain. No abnormal clinical signs were seen. Haemoglobin and haematocrit values were not affected by the treatment, but there were marginal effects on mean erythrocyte volume in some treated groups. Male rats fed 50 or 250 mg/kg showed decreased plasma triglyceride levels and a dose-related increase in hepatic APDM activity. The latter effect was also seen in females fed 250 mg/kg. Small increases in urinary glucose excretion occurred in males fed 50 or 250 mg/kg after 13 weeks. No treatment-related effects on organ weights and no significant histopathological changes were reported (Lindsay et al., 1981).

In studies by Lindsay et al. (1982), two groups of 32 male rats were fed either a control diet or a diet containing 250 mg cyhalothrin/kg for 28 days. After this period eight rats per group were killed and examined. The remaining rats were fed the control diet for periods of 7, 14, or 28 days after cessation of treatment, and a further eight rats per group were killed and examined at each of these time intervals. A decrease in body weight gain was seen in the treated rats, which, although not statistically significant, was still much reduced at the end of the 28-day recovery period. Proliferation of the hepatic smooth endoplasmic reticulum and elevated hepatic APDM activity were also seen in the treated animals. These effects had reversed 7 days after the cessation of treatment with cyhalothrin and were considered to be physiological adaptive changes rather than a toxicological effect.

When groups of 20 male and 20 female Alderley Park rats received diets containing 0, 10, 50, or 250 mg lambda-cyhalothrin/kg for 90 days, decreased body weight gain, accompanied by a reduction in food consumption, was seen in both male and female rats receiving the highest dose. No abnormal clinical signs were seen; in particular, there was no evidence of neurological effects. There were no treatment-related effects on haematological parameters but reductions in the activities of plasma alanine transaminase (males only) and alkaline phosphatase (females only at 13 weeks) were apparent in animals fed the highest dose. Plasma triglycerides were also reduced in males at this feeding level. Relative liver weights were increased in both sexes at 250 mg/kg and in males at 50 mg/kg, accompanied by increased activity of hepatic APDM. No other changes in organ weight or histopathology were attributed to treatment with lambda-cyhalothrin. These two effects, particularly in view of the findings with cyhalothrin, were considered to be adaptive in nature and the toxicological NOEL was established at 50 mg/kg (equivalent to 2.5 mg/kg body weight per day (Hart et al., 1985).

7.3.1.2 Dog

In studies by Chesterman et al. (1980), groups of one male and one female dog (Alderley Park beagles) received 0, 2.5, or 10 mg cyhalothrin/kg body weight orally in corn oil by gelatine capsule daily for four weeks. A further group initially received 30 mg/kg per day, but due to severe clinical signs after 10 days dosing, which were typical of pyrethroid toxicity (muscular trembling, unsteadiness, vomiting, and body weight loss), the animals were rested and then received 20 mg/kg per day for four weeks. Similar clinical signs were seen, with the exception of body weight loss, in all animals receiving 10 mg/kg per day or more, the severity being dose related. Investigation of the sciatic and tibial nerves and the lumbricalis muscle with special histopathological stains indicated no changes that could be attributed to treatment with cyhalothrin. Liquid faeces were produced by all animals receiving cyhalothrin, the incidence being dose related. These changes were considered to be of no toxicological significance. No other changes were observed that could be attributed to the treatment.

When groups of 6 male and 6 female dogs (Alderley Park beagles) were fed cyhalothrin in corn oil by gelatine capsule at 0, 1, 2.5, or 10 mg/kg body weight per day for 26 weeks, signs of pyrethroid toxicity were seen in some dogs at 10 mg/kg. Although liquid faeces were produced by all animals in the study, including the controls, the incidence and frequency were higher in treated animals and were dose related. These changes were considered to be of no toxicological significance. Macroscopic postmortem examination, organ weights, and histological investigations revealed no treatment-related changes. The oral NOEL in dogs was found to be 2.5 mg/kg per day (Chesterman et al., 1981).

In studies by Hext et al. (1986), groups of 6 male and 6 female dogs were dosed by gavage in corn oil with 0, 0.1, 0.5, or 3.5 mg lambda-cyhalothrin/kg body weight daily for 52 weeks. Clinical signs of neurological effects were evident in all animals fed the highest dose, which were unaccompanied by histological changes in the nervous system. There was an increased incidence of fluid faeces at the highest dose and a slight increase in the group receiving 0.5 mg/kg per day. This effect was considered to be related to the method of administration and not to be toxicologically significant. No histopathological changes attributable to lambda-cyhalothrin administration were observed at any of the dose levels employed, and the toxicological NOEL in this study was 0.5 mg lambda-cyhalothrin per kg per day.

7.3.2 Dermal

7.3.2.1 Rabbit

Cyhalothrin in polyethylene glycol (PEG 300) (10, 100, or 1000 mg/kg body weight per day) was applied to the skin of groups of 10 male and 10 female New Zealand White rabbits and kept in contact with the skin 6 h/day, 5 days per week for 3 weeks (i.e. a total of 15 applications) by means of an occlusive dressing. A group of 14 male and 14 female control rabbits was treated with polyethylene glycol (PEG 300) using the same procedure. The skin of half the animals in each group was abraded prior to the application of cyhalothrin. Repeated application of the vehicle alone (polyethylene glycol) and the vehicle plus cyhalothrin caused slight to severe skin irritation. At the highest dose level there was an increased incidence of oedema and erythema. A small number of animals given the highest dose showed pyrethroid-like symptoms, but only when the skin was unabraded. The NOEL was considered to be 100 mg/kg per day (Henderson & Jackson, 1982).

7.4 Long-term exposures and carcinogenicity

7.4.1 Rat

In studies by Pigott et al. (1984), groups of 72 male and 72 female Alpk/AP strain rats were fed diets containing cyhalothrin at levels of 0, 10, 50, or 250 mg/kg diet for up to 104 weeks. All the surviving animals were sacrificed, and histopathological and gross postmortem examinations were carried out. Decreased body weight gain, accompanied by a small decrease in food consumption, was evident in rats of both sexes fed the highest dose. This was accompanied by minor changes in blood biochemistry. Increased liver weight was seen in rats of both sexes fed cyhalothrin at 250 mg/kg at the interim sacrifice but this was not evident at termination. There was no histopathological evidence of a chronic toxic effect due to cyhalothrin. In particular clinical and histopathological evaluation gave no indication of an effect on the nervous system. There was no evidence for a carcinogenic effect of cyhalothrin. The toxicological NOEL for this study was 50 mg cyhalothrin/kg diet, corresponding to a minimum dose rate of approximately 1.7 mg/kg body weight per day for male rats and 1.9 mg/kg per day for female rats.

7.4.2 Mouse

Groups of 52 male and 52 female Charles River CD-1 mice were maintained for 104 weeks on diets containing 0, 20, 100, or 500 mg cyhalothrin/kg and further groups of 12 males and 12 females were designated for interim sacrifice after 52 weeks. During the study there were no deaths attributable to treatment with cyhalothrin. Signs of toxicity ascribable to cyhalothrin included piloerection and hunched posture in both sexes at 500 mg/kg and in males at 100 mg/kg and reduced body weight gain, higher food intake, and reduced efficiency of food utilization in males receiving 500 mg/kg. There was a statistically significant increase, compared to the controls, in the incidence of mammary adenocarcinoma in females at the two highest dose levels. However, the frequency of these tumours was not unduly at variance with that normally seen in the strain of mouse used, and no dose relationship was apparent. Thus, there were no neoplastic findings that could be attributed to the long-term administration of cyhalothrin. There was a clear NOEL of 20 mg/kg, corresponding to a mean calculated daily intake of 1.8 mg/kg body weight per day in males and 2.0 mg/kg body weight per day in females (Colley et al., 1984).

7.5 Reproduction, embryotoxicity, and teratogenicity

7.5.1 Reproduction

In studies by Milburn et al. (1984), groups of 15 male and 30 female (F_0 parents) weaning Alderley Park rats were fed diets containing 0, 10, 30, or 100 mg cyhalothrin per kg. After 12 weeks, the animals were mated to produce the first (F_{1a}) litter and subsequently re-mated to produce a second (F_{1b}) litter. The breeding programme was repeated with F_1 parents selected from the F_{1b} offspring and F_2 parents selected from the F_{2b} offspring. Test diets were fed continuously throughout the study. There were minor effects on body weight gain of parents from all generations receiving 100 mg/kg, but no clinical signs of neurological effects were seen in either parents or offspring. No effects of treatment were seen on indices of male and female fertility, gestation period, live born index, or pup survival. There was a small reduction in mean total litter weight of the F_2 and F_3 generations from rats receiving the highest dose, which was attributable to minor decreases in litter size and a small reduction in weight gain of the pups. No effect was seen in litters from rats receiving 30 mg/kg. There was no evidence of gross or histopathological change attributable to the treatment. The reproductive effects seen in rats receiving the highest dose were of a minor nature. A clear NOEL of 30 mg/kg (corresponding to a dosage in the range of 1.5 to 1.9 mg/kg body weight per day) was established (Milburn et al., 1984).

7.5.2 Embryotoxicity and teratogenicity

7.5.2.1 Rat

When groups of 24 mated female rats (Charles River CD-1) were given cyhalothrin orally (in corn oil), at 0, 5, 10, or 15 mg/kg body weight per day, from day 6 to 15 inclusive of gestation and were killed on day 20, there was reduced body weight gain at the highest dose level and evidence of mild pyrethroid toxicity in two of these animals. There were no other effects on the clinical or litter parameters attributable to treatment with cyhalothrin, and examination of the viscera and skeletons showed no effects of treatment. At the highest dose level, there was maternal toxicity, but there was no effect on any aspect of fetal development at any dose level (Killick, 1981a).

7.5.2.2 Rabbit

In studies by Killick (1981b), groups of at least 18 pregnant New Zealand White rabbits received cyhalothrin orally in corn oil daily at 0, 3, 10, or 30 mg/kg body weight, from days 6 to 18 (inclusive) of gestation and were killed on day 28. There was reduced body weight gain at the highest dose, accompanied by reduced food intake during dosing. There were no clinical signs and no changes in pregnancy incidence or in litter parameters attributable to treatment with cyhalothrin. Examination of the viscera and skeletons revealed no effects of treatment. At the highest dose level, there was maternal toxicity, but there was no effect on any aspect of fetal development at any dose level.

7.6 Mutagenicity and related end-points

7.6.1 Microorganisms

Five test strains, TA1535, TA1537, TA1538, TA98, and TA100, were employed to evaluate the mutagenic potential of cyhalothrin using the salmonella reverse mutation assay of Ames. The assay was conducted in the presence and absence of metabolic activation (S9 mix) with cyhalothrin at levels up to 2500 μg/plate. The mean numbers of revertant colonies of Salmonella typhimurium observed in the five test strains indicated an unequivocal negative response (Trueman, 1981). Lambda-cyhalothrin at dose levels of up to 5000 μg/plate, both in the presence and absence of metabolic activation, gave a non-mutagenic response in the same test using the same strains (Callander, 1984).

7.6.2 In vitro mammalian cells

When cyhalothrin was tested in a modification of the cell culture transformation test of Styles, using Syrian Hamster kidney cell line BHK21C13, the response in the presence of metabolic activation was unequivocally negative. In the absence of metabolic transformation there was an erratic increase in numbers of transformed colonies together with a poor dose response. These data were not thought to indicate a significant positive response, and it was concluded that cyhalothrin does not appear to possess significant cell-transforming properties (Richold et al., 1981). In addition, the significance of the results from the BHK cell system is doubtful in view of the questionable interlaboratory reproducibility of this assay.

The mutagenic potential of lambda-cyhalothrin has been assessed *in vitro* with L51787 mouse lymphoma cells, both in the presence and absence of auxiliary metabolic activation (S9) mix, using dose levels of 125-1000, 2000, and 4000 μg/ml. There was no increase in mutation frequency either in the presence or absence of S9 mix (Cross, 1985).

Lambda-cyhalothrin, at dose levels of up to 1000 μg/ml, either in the presence or absence of metabolic activation, did not induce statistically significant increases in the incorporation of tritiated thymidine in cultured human (Hela) cells (Milone, 1986) or induce chromosomal damage in human lymphocytes stimulated by phytohaemagglutinin (Sheldon et al., 1985).

7.6.3 *In vivo* mammalian assays

Male rats were given a single dose or five consecutive daily doses by gavage of cyhalothrin at levels of 1.5, 7.5, or 15 mg/kg, and bone marrow samples were taken and examined for chromosomal abnormalities. The results indicated that cyhalothrin has no clastogenic potential (Anderson et al., 1981).

In studies by Irvine (1981), three groups of male mice were dosed with cyhalothrin by gavage, at dose levels of 1, 5, or 10 mg/kg daily, for 5 consecutive days. A further group received the known mutagen cyclophosphamide intraperitoneally at 200 mg/kg daily for five days. The animals were then mated with groups of females at weekly intervals for eight weeks. Pregnancy incidence, pre- and post-implantation loss, clinical condition, body weight, and gross necropsy were assessed. There was no evidence of an increase in the dominant lethal mutation frequency following treatment. The NOEL was 10 mg/kg per day. Although these studies showed no clastogenic or mutagenic effect, it is not clear whether sufficiently high dose levels were used.

When lambda-cyhalothrin was administered to mice at levels of up to 35 mg/kg and bone marrow preparations were examined for the formation of micronuclei in polychromatic erythrocytes, there was no statistically significant increase in the frequency of micronuclei, compared to control animals. The positive control substance, cyclophosphamide, showed the expected response (Sheldon et al., 1984).

7.7 Mode of action

The mode of action of cyhalothrin and lambda-cyhalothrin, both type II pyrethroids, is basically the same as that of the other pyrethroids (see Appendix).

8. EFFECTS ON HUMANS

8.1 General population exposure

No poisoning incidents with cyhalothrin or lambda-cyhalothrin have been reported. There is no information on effects from short- or long-term exposure and no epidemiological information is available.

8.2 Occupational exposure

Cyhalothrin is known to produce an effect described as subjective facial sensation (SFS) in some people working with this compound. SFS is a transient phenomenon; symptoms are not associated with objective physical signs and recovery appears to be complete. It is likely that SFS arises from direct facial contact with the chemical particularly from touching the face with contaminated gloves or hands. This would also help to explain the effect of formulation or concentration as these could affect the rate of dermal penetration and therefore access of the chemical to the nerve endings.

It appears unlikely that individual sensitivity is important in the development of symptoms following exposure. It is more likely to be related to the amount of the chemical that comes into contact with the facial skin. The information currently available (Hart, 1984) is summarized in section 8.2.2.

8.2.1 Acute toxicity: poisoning incidents

No poisoning incidents involving cyhalothrin or lambda-cyhalothrin have been reported.

8.2.2 Effects of short- and long-term exposure

Laboratory workers and manufacturing plant and field operators handling natural and synthetic pyrethroids, including cyhalothrin and lambda-cyhalothrin, have noticed a transient skin sensation in the periorbital area of the face and other sites after direct skin exposure. It has been suggested that these sensations are caused by spontaneous repetitive firing of sensory nerve fibres or nerve endings, whose threshold has been transiently lowered by the compound, localized around the sites of exposure.

Symptoms from exposure to a synthetic pyrethroid generally start 30 min to 1 h after exposure and last for several hours, sometimes up to 2 days. They almost always affect the facial area, producing a tingling, burning, or numb sensation that has been variously described as paraesthesia, dysaesthesia, or SFS. The latter term appears most appropriate as no objective signs of abnormality of nerve function have been found in workers suffering from these effects and the facial area is by far the most commonly affected.

8.2.2.1 *Manufacture*

At least 12 workers involved in the manufacture of cyhalothrin have experienced symptoms of SFS. The symptoms were described as burning, tingling, or sunburn, but clinical examination revealed no abnormal neurological signs. The areas of the face affected were the eyelids, cheeks, nostrils, forehead, and lips. In one case the penis was affected, probably from contact with contaminated hands. The symptoms started between 5 min and 3 h from the onset of exposure and lasted from 5 to 30 h. Wind, washing, and temperature increase led to a worsening of the symptoms, and relief could be obtained by using a local anaesthetic. Barrier creams were relatively ineffective in preventing the symptoms.

8.2.2.2 *Formulation and laboratory work*

Two workers have been reported to have suffered from SFS. Both were exposed to technical cyhalothrin and symptoms began 1-6 h after exposure. The symptoms described were typical of SFS, consisting of tingling and burning around the eyes and facial area, and lasted 6-24 h.

Four reports involving three individuals have been received from laboratories involved with lambda-cyhalothrin. The symptoms consisted of a facial tingling and burning sensation and in one case tingling on the tongue. Symptoms began within 30 min of exposure and lasted from

6 h to 2 days. All three workers were involved in handling either technical material or concentrated lambda-cyhalothrin solutions (10% w/v ai).

8.2.2.3 *Field use*

Virtually no reports have been received on the agricultural or public health use of cyhalothrin. The only information that has become available is from the use of cyhalothrin in animal health products. Skin itching has been reported following exposure to a 5% emulsifiable concentrate of cyhalothrin, but dilutions of 0.1% and 0.005% (w/v of ai) were without significant effect. More recently, several incidents of facial irritation have been reported following the use of cyhalothrin in sheep sprays (Hart, 1984). The concentration used in these sprays was very low (0.002% w/v), but the characteristics of the spray used were unclear.

Out of 38 field trials staff who returned questionnaires, only four reported experiencing any adverse effects as a result of exposure to lambda-cyhalothrin. Three of these individuals experienced a burning sensation or irritation around the face, cheeks, or eyes, which started between 45 and 60 min after initial exposure and lasted, respectively, for 5, 18, and 72 h. In one case the symptoms were severe enough to prevent the individual from working. The other field trials worker experienced a rash on the hands that started 24 h after exposure and lasted several days. All four field trials staff were involved in handling concentrated solutions of lambda-cyhalothrin (2.5% w/v ai) and three of the four sprayed diluted solutions. None of the three workers experiencing the facial sensation had experienced similar symptoms before, but the worker who developed the rash had suffered a similar rash after exposure to permethrin, cypermethrin, and deltamethrin following their application to top fruit. Eight of the other 34 field trials staff returning questionnaires stated that they had previously suffered symptoms of facial tingling or burning.

9. PREVIOUS EVALUATIONS BY INTERNATIONAL BODIES

Cyhalothrin was discussed at the 1984 and 1986 FAO/WHO Joint Meetings on Pesticide Residues (JMPR), where an acceptable daily intake (ADI) for cyhalothrin of 0-0.02 mg/kg body weight was established (FAO/WHO, 1985, 1986a).

The JMPR (FAO/WHO, 1985, 1986a,b) has estimated maximum residue limits (MRLs) for cyhalothrin (sum of the isomers) as follows:

Commodity	Maximum residue limit	Pre-harvest interval (days)
Pome fruits	0.2	14
Cabbages, head	0.2	3-4
Potatoes	0.02[a]	non specified
Cotton seed	0.02[a]	21
Cotton seed oil, crude	0.02[a]	non specified
Cotton seed oil, edible	0.02[a]	non specified

[a] At or about the limit of detection.

REFERENCES

ANDERSON, D., RICHARDSON, C.R., HULME, A., MORRIS, J., BANHAM, P.B., & GODLEY, M.J. (1981) *Cyhalothrin: A cytogenic study in the rat* (Unpublished proprietary report No. CTL/P/664, submitted to WHO by ICI).

BARBER, J.E. (1985) *PP321: Acute dermal toxicity study* (Unpublished proprietary report No. CTL/P/1119, submitted to WHO by ICI).

BENGSTONE, M., DAVIES, R.A.H., DESMARCHELIER, J.M., HENNING, R., MURRAY, W., SIMPSON, B.W., SNELSON, J.T., STICKA, R., & WALLBANK, B.E. (1983) Organophosphorothioates and synergised synthetic pyrethroids as grain protectants on bulk wheat. *Pestic. Sci.*, **14**: 373-384.

BEWICK, D.W. & ZINNER, C.K.J. (1981) *Cyhalothrin: Degradation in soil* (Unpublished proprietary report No. RJ0203B, submitted to WHO by ICI).

BHARTI, H. & BEWICK, D.W. (1986) *Cyhalothrin: Degradation in a Japanese soil* (Unpublished proprietary report No. RJ0491B, submitted to WHO by ICI).

BHARTI, H., BEWICK, D.W., & WHITE, R.D. (1985) *PP563 and PP321: Degradation in soil* (Unpublished proprietary report No. RJ0382B, submitted to WHO by ICI).

CALLANDER, R.D. (1984) *PP321: An evaluation in the Salmonella mutagenicity assay* (Unpublished proprietary report No. CTL/P/1000, submitted to WHO by ICI).

CHESTERMAN, H., HEYWOOD, R., ALLEN, T.R., STREET, A.E., PRENTICE, D., BUCKLEY, P., & OFFER, J. (1980) *PP563: Preliminary oral toxicity study in beagle dogs* (Unpublished proprietary report of the Huntingdon Research Centre No. 325/8074, submitted to WHO by ICI).

CHESTERMAN, H., HAYWOOD, R., ALLEN, T.R., STREET, A.E., KELLY, D.F., GOPINATH, C., & PRENTICE, D.E. (1981) *Cyhalothrin oral toxicity study in beagle dogs (Final report: Repeated daily dosing for 26 weeks)* (Unpublished proprietary report of the Huntingdon Research Centre No. ICI/326/8162, submitted to WHO by ICI).

COLLEY, J., DAWE, S., HEYWOOD, R., ALMOND, R., GIBSON, W.A., GREGSON, R., & GOPINATH, C. (1984) *Cyhalothrin potential tumorigenic and toxic effects in prolonged dietary administration to mice* (Unpublished proprietary report of the Huntingdon Research Centre No. ICI 395/83668, submitted to WHO by ICI).

COLLIS, W.M.D. & LEAHEY, J.P. (1984) *PP321: Hydrolysis in water at pH 5, 7 and 9* (Unpublished proprietary report No. RJ0338B, submitted to WHO by ICI).

COULSON, J.M., COLLINS, I.G., & EDWARDS, P.J. (1986) *PP321: Effects on earthworms Lumbricidae of repeated annual field applications* (Unpublished proprietary report No. RJ0511B, submitted to WHO by ICI).

CROSS, M. (1985) *PP321: Assessment of mutagenic potential using L5178Y mouse lymphoma cells* (Unpublished proprietary report No. CTL/P/1340, submitted to WHO by ICI).

CROSSLAND, N.O. (1982) Aquatic toxicology of cypermethrin. II. Fate and biological effects in pond experiments. *Aquat. Toxicol.*, **2**: 205-222.

CROSSLAND, N.O., SHIRES, S.W., & BENNETT, D. (1982) Aquatic toxicology of cypermethrin. III. Fate and biological effects of spray drift deposits in freshwater adjacent to agricultural land. *Aquat. Toxicol.*, **2**: 253-270.

CURL, E.A., LEAHEY, J.P., & LLOYD, S.J. (1984a) *PP321: Aqueous photolysis at pH 5* (Unpublished proprietary report No. RJ0362B, submitted to WHO by ICI).

CURL, E.A., LEAHEY, J.P., & LLOYD, D. (1984b) *PP321: Photodegradation on a soil surface* (Unpublished proprietary report No. RJ0358B, submitted to WHO by ICI).

ELLIOTT, M. (1977) *Synthetic pyrethroids*, Washington, DC, American Chemical Society, pp. 229 (ACS Symposium Series 42).

EVANS, M.H. (1976) End-plate potentials in frog muscle exposed to a synthetic pyrethroid. *Pestic. Biochem. Physiol.*, **6**: 547-550.

FAO (1982) *Report of the Second Government Consultation on International Harmonization of Pesticide Registration Requirements, Rome, 11-15 October*, Rome, Food and Agriculture Organization of the United Nations.

FAO/WHO (1985) Cyhalothrin. In: *1984 Evaluations of some pesticide residues in food*, Rome, Food and Agricultural Organization of the United Nations, pp. 173-185, 571-584 (FAO Plant production and protection Paper 67).

FAO/WHO (1986a) Cyhalothrin: In: *1986 Evaluations of some pesticide residues in food, Part 1: Residues*, Rome, Food and Agriculture Organization of the United Nations, pp. 95-138 (FAO Plant Production and Protection Paper 78).

FAO/WHO (1986b) *Codex maximum limits for pesticide residues*, 2nd ed., Rome, Codex Alimentarius Commission, Food and Agriculture Organization of the United Nations (CAC XIII).

FARRELLY, E., HAMER, M.J., & HILL, I.R. (1984) *PP321: Toxicity to first instar* Daphnia magna (Unpublished proprietary report No. RJ0359B, submitted to WHO by ICI).

FARRELLY, E., HAMER, M.J., & HILL, I.R. (1985) *PP321: Toxicity of formulations JF9509 and GFU383C to first instar* Daphnia magna (Unpublished proprietary report No. RJ0426B, submitted to WHO by ICI).

FITZPATRICK, R.D. (1985) *PP321 dissipation in US soils - 1983* (Unpublished report No. TMU1809, submitted to WHO by ICI).

FLANNIGAN, S.A. & TUCKER, S.B. (1985) Variation in cutaneous sensation between synthetic pyrethroid insecticides. *Contact dermatitis*, **13**: 140-147.

FORBES, S. & DUTTON, A.J. (1985) A small scale method for the determination of pyrethroid insecticide residues in crops and soils. *Pestic. Sci.*, **16**: 404-408.

GAMMON, D.W. & CASIDA, J.E. (1983) Pyrethroids of the most potent class antagonize GABA action at the crayfish neuromuscular junction. *Neurosci. Lett.*, **40**: 163-168.

GAMMON, D.W., BROWN, M.A., & CASIDA, J.E. (1981) Two classes of pyrethroid action in the cockroach. *Pestic. Biochem. Physiol.*, **15**: 181-191.

GAMMON, D.W., LAWRENCE, L.J., & CASIDA, J.E. (1982) Pyrethroid toxicology: Protective effects of Diazepam and phenobarbital in the mouse and the cockroach. *Toxicol. appl. Pharmacol.*, **66**: 290-296.

GIFAP (1981) *Technical Monograph No. 4: Guidelines on pesticide residue trials to provide residue data for the registration of pesticides and the establishment of maximum residue limits*, Brussels, International Group of National Associations of Manufacturers of Agrochemical Products (GIFAP D/1981/2537/3).

GIRENKO, D.B. & KLISENKO, M.A. (1984) Concentration and determination of trace quantities of synthetic pyrethroids in the air. *Gig. i Sanit.*, **3**: 57-59.

GLICKMAN, A.H. & CASIDA, J.E. (1982) Species and structural variations affecting pyrethroid neurotoxicity. *Neurobehav. Toxicol. Teratol.*, **4**(6): 793-799.

GOUGH, H.J., COLLINS, I.G., EVERETT, C.J., & WILKINSON, W. (1984) *PP321: Acute contact and oral toxicity to honey bees* (Apis mellifera) (Unpublished proprietary report No. RJ0390B, submitted to WHO by ICI).

GOUGH, H.J., COLLINS, I.G., & WILKINSON, W. (1985) *PP321: Field test of toxicity to honey bees* (Apis mellifera) *on flowering oil-seed rape* (Brassica napus) (Unpublished proprietary report No. RJ0413B, submitted to WHO by ICI).

HALL, J.S. & LEAHEY, J.P. (1983) *Cyhalothrin: Fate in river water* (Unpublished proprietary report No. RJ0320B, submitted to WHO by ICI).

HAMER, M.J. & HILL, I.R. (1985) *Cyhalothrin: The accumulation of cyhalothrin and its degradation products by channel catfish and* Daphnia magna *in a soil/water system* (Unpublished proprietary report No. RJ0427B, submitted to WHO by ICI).

HAMER, M.J., FARRELLY, E., & HILL, I.R. (1985a) *PP321: Toxicity to* Gammarus pulex (Unpublished proprietary report No. RJ0414B, submitted to WHO by ICI).

HAMER, M.J., FARRELLY, E., & HILL, I.R. (1985b) *PP321: 21 day* Daphnia magna *life-cycle study* (Unpublished proprietary report No. RJ0451B, submitted to WHO by ICI).

HARRISON, M.P. (1981) *Cyhalothrin: The disposition and metabolism of [^{14}C]-146814 in rats* (Unpublished proprietary report No. 10/HD/007325, submitted to WHO by ICI).

HARRISON, M.P. (1983) *Cyhalothrin: The metabolism and disposition of 146814 in the rat: Part IV. Isolation and identification of the major urinary metabolites derived from [^{14}C-benzyl]- or [^{14}C-cyclopropyl]-146814 following oral administration* (Unpublished proprietary report No. 6/HC/005683, submitted to WHO by ICI).

HARRISON, M.P. (1984a) *Cyhalothrin (146814): The metabolism and disposition of 146814 in rats: Part II. Tissue residues derived from [^{14}C-benzyl] or [^{14}C-cyclopropyl]-146814, after a single oral dose of 1 or 25 mg/kg* (Unpublished proprietary report No. KMR 002/2, submitted to WHO by ICI).

HARRISON, M.P. (1984b) *Cyhalothrin: The metabolism and disposition of [^{14}C]-146814 in rats: Part III. Studies to determine radioactive residues in the rat following 14 days repeated oral administration* (Unpublished proprietary report No. 146814 KMR 002/03, submitted to WHO by ICI).

HARRISON, M.P. (1984c) *Cyhalothrin (146814): The disposition and metabolism of [^{14}C]-146814 in the dog* (Unpublished proprietary report No. 146814 KMD 005, submitted to WHO by ICI).

HARRISON, M.P. (1984d) *Cyhalothrin (146814): The metabolism, excretion and residues in the cow after 7 days oral administration with two [^{14}C]-labelled forms of 146814 at 1 mg/kg/day* (Unpublished proprietary report No. 146814 KMC 006/007, submitted to WHO by ICI).

HART, D., BANHAM, P.B., CHART, I.S., EVANS, D.P., GORE, C.W., STONARD, M.D., MORELAND, S., GODLEY, M.J., & ROBINSON, M. (1985) *PP321: 90-day feeding study in rats* (Unpublished proprietary report No. CTL/P/1045, submitted to WHO by ICI).

HART, T.B. (1984) *Review of adverse skin reactions associated with the use of synthetic pyrethroids* (Unpublished proprietary report No. TMF2530, submitted to WHO by ICI).

HENDERSON, C. & JACKSON, S.J. (1982) *Cyhalothrin: Subacute dermal toxicity study in rabbits* (Unpublished proprietary report No. CTL/P/680, submitted to WHO by ICI).

HEXT, P.M., BRAMMER, A., CHALMERS, D.T., CHART, I.S., GORE, C.W., PATE, I., & BANHAM, P.B. (1986) *PP321: 1 year oral dosing study in dogs* (Unpublished proprietary report No. CTL/P/1316, submitted to WHO by ICI).

HILL, R.W. (1981) *Determination of the acute toxicity of cyhalothrin (PP563) to Rainbow trout* (Salmo gairdneri) (Unpublished proprietary report No. BL/B/2097, submitted to WHO by ICI).

HILL, R.W. (1984a) *PP321: Determination of acute toxicity to Rainbow trout* (Salmo gairdneri) (Unpublished proprietary report No. BL/B/2405, submitted to WHO by ICI).

HILL, R.W. (1984b) *PP321: Determination of acute toxicity to Bluegill sunfish* (Lepomis macrochirus) (Unpublished proprietary report No. BL/B/2406, submitted to WHO by ICI).

HILL, R.W. (1985a) *PP321: Determination of acute toxicity to Rainbow trout* (Salmo gairdneri) *of 2.5% w/w formulation* (Unpublished proprietary report No. BL/B/2603, submitted to WHO by ICI).

HILL, R.W. (1985b) *PP321: Determination of acute toxicity of a 1 lb/US gallon EC formulation to Rainbow trout* (Salmo gairdneri) (Unpublished proprietary report No. BL/B/2609, submitted to WHO by ICI).

HILL, R.W. (1985c) *PP321: Determination of acute toxicity to Rainbow trout* (Salmo gairdneri) *of a 5% EC formulation* (Unpublished proprietary report No. BL/B/2783, submitted to WHO by ICI).

HILL, R.W. (1985d) *PP321: Determination of acute toxicity to Mirror carp* (Cyprinus carpio) *of a 2.5% w/w formulation* (Unpublished proprietary report No. BL/B/2604, submitted to WHO by ICI).

HILL, R.W. (1985e) *PP321: Determination of acute toxicity to Mirror carp* (Cyprinus carpio) *of a 5% EC formulation* (Unpublished proprietary report No. BL/B/2784, submitted to WHO by ICI).

HILL, R.W. (1985f) *PP321: Determination of acute toxicity of a 1 lb/US gallon EC formulation to Bluegill sunfish* (Lepomis macrochirus) (Unpublished proprietary report No. BL/B/2610, submitted to WHO by ICI).

HILL, R.W. (1985g) *PP321: Determination of acute toxicity to Sheepshead minnow* (Cyprinodon variegatus) (Unpublished proprietary report No. BL/B/2615, submitted to WHO by ICI).

HILL, R.W., CAUNTER, J.E., & CUMMING, R.I. (1985) *PP321: Determination of the chronic toxicity to Sheepshead minnow* (Cyprinodon variegatus) *embryos and larvae* (Unpublished proprietary report No. BL/B/2677, submitted to WHO by ICI).

IRVINE, L.F.H. (1981) *Cyhalothrin: Oral (gavage) dominant lethal study in the male mouse* (Unpublished proprietary report of the Hazleton Laboratories No. 2647-72/213, submitted to WHO by ICI).

JACKSON, S.J. (1981) *Cyhalothrin: Eye irritation study in the rabbit* (Unpublished proprietary report No. CTL/T/1502, submitted to WHO by ICI).

JACKSON, S.J. & NIXON, J. (1981) *Cyhalothrin: Skin irritation studies in the rabbit and rat* (Unpublished proprietary report No. CTL/T/1504, submitted to WHO by ICI).

KILLICK, M.E. (1981a) *Cyhalothrin: Oral (gavage) teratology study in the rat* (Unpublished proprietary report of the Hazleton Laboratories No. 2661-72/208, submitted to WHO by ICI).

KILLICK, M.E. (1981b) *Cyhalothrin: Oral (gavage) teratology study in the New Zealand white rabbit* (Unpublished proprietary report of the Hazleton Laboratories No. 2700-72/211, submitted to WHO by ICI).

LAWRENCE, L.J. & CASIDA, J.E. (1982) Pyrethroid toxicology: Mouse intracerebral structure-toxicity relationship. *Pestic. Biochem. Physiol.*, **18**: 9-14.

LAWRENCE, L.J. & CASIDA, J.E. (1983) Stereospecific action of pyrethroid insecticides on the gamma-aminobutyric acid receptor-ionophore complex. *Science*, **221**: 1399-1401.

LAWRENCE, L.J., GEE, K.W., & YAMAMURA, H.I. (1985) Interactions of pyrethroid insecticides with chloride ionophore-associated binding sites. *Neurotoxicology*, **6**: 87-98.

LEAHEY, J.P. (1985) *The pyrethroid insecticides*, London, Taylor & Francis Ltd, 440 pp.

LEAHEY, J.P. & FRENCH, D.A. (1986a) *Quantification and characterisation of radioactive residues found in soya leaves from plants treated with ^{14}C-PP321* (Unpublished proprietary report No. RJ0507B, submitted to WHO by ICI).

LEAHEY, J.P. & FRENCH, D.A. (1986b) *Quantification and characterisation of radioactive residues found in cotton leaves from plants treated with ^{14}C-cyclopropane-labelled PP321* (Unpublished proprietary report No. JR0526B, submitted to WHO by ICI).

LEAHEY, J.P. & FRENCH, D.A. (1986c) *Quantification and characterisation of radioactive residues in cotton leaves from plants treated ^{14}C-benzyl-labelled PP321* (Unpublished proprietary report No. RJ0497B, submitted to WHO by ICI).

LEAHEY, J.P. & PARKER, S. (1985) *Cyhalothrin: Characterisation of residues accumulated by carp continuously exposed to ^{14}C-cyhalothrin* (Unpublished proprietary report No. RJ0407B, submitted to WHO by ICI).

LEAHEY, J.P., FRENCH, D.A., & HEATH, J. (1985) *PP321: Metabolism in a goat* (Unpublished proprietary Report No. RJ0435B, submitted to WHO by ICI).

LINDSAY, S., CHART, I.S., GODLEY, M.J., GORE, C.W., HALL, M., PRATT, I., ROBINSON, M., & STONARD, M. (1981) *Cyhalothrin: 90-day feeding study in rats* (Unpublished proprietary report No. CTL/P/629, submitted to WHO by ICI).

LINDSAY, S., DOE, J.E., GODLEY, M.J., HALL, M., PRATT, I., ROBINSON, M., & STONARD, M.D. (1982) *Cyhalothrin induced liver changes: Reversibility study in male rats* (Unpublished proprietary report No. CTL/P/668, submitted to WHO by ICI).

LUND, A.E. & NARAHASHI, T. (1983) Kinetics of sodium channel modification as the basis for the variation in the nerve membrane effects of pyrethroids and DDT analogs. *Pestic. Biochem. Physiol.*, **20**: 203-216.

MILBURN, G.M., BANHAM, P., GODLEY, M.J., PIGOTT, G., & ROBINSON, M. (1984) *Cyhalothrin: Three generation reproduction study in the rat* (Unpublished proprietary report No. CTL/P/906, submitted to WHO by ICI).

MILONE, M.F. (1986) *PP321: Unscheduled DNA synthesis in cultured Hela cells (autoradiographic method)* (Unpublished proprietary report of the Institute di Ricerche Biomediche Antione Marxer No. M914, submitted to WHO by ICI).

MIYAMOTO, J. (1981) The chemistry, metabolism and residue analysis of synthetic pyrethroids. *Pure appl. Chem.*, **53**: 1967-2922.

MIYAMOTO, J. & KEARNEY, P.C. (1983) *Pesticide chemistry-human welfare and the environment. Proceedings of the Fifth International Congress on Pesticide Chemistry, Kyoto, Japan, 29 August-4 September, 1982*, Oxford, New York, Pergamon Press (Vol. 1-4).

NIXON, J. & JACKSON, S.J. (1981a) *Cyhalothrin: Acute toxicity* (Unpublished proprietary report No. CTL/T/1555, submitted to WHO by ICI).

NIXON, J. & JACKSON, S.J. (1981b) *Cyhalothrin: Skin sensitisation study in the guinea-pig* (Unpublished proprietary report No. CTL/T/1552, submitted to WHO by ICI).

PIGOTT, G.H., CHART, I.S., GODLEY, M.J., GORE, C.W., HOLLIS, K.J., ROBINSON, M., TAYLOR, K., & TINSTON, D.J. (1984) *Cyhalothrin: Two year feeding study in rats* (Unpublished proprietary report No. CTL/P/980, submitted to WHO by ICI).

PRITCHARD, V.K. (1984) *PP321: Skin sensitisation study* (Unpublished proprietary report No. CTL/P/1054, submitted to WHO by ICI).

PRITCHARD, V.K. (1985a) *PP321 and cyhalothrin: skin irritation study* (Unpublished proprietary report No. CTL/P/1139, submitted to WHO by ICI).

PRITCHARD, V.K. (1985b) *PP321: Eye irritation study* (Unpublished proprietary report No. CTL/P/1207, submitted to WHO by ICI).

PROUT, M.S. (1984) *Cyhalothrin: Bioaccumulation in the rat* (Unpublished proprietary report No. CTL/P/1014, submitted to WHO by ICI).

PROUT, M.S., & HOWARD, E.F. (1985) *PP321: Comparative absorption study in the rat (1 mg/kg)* (Unpublished proprietary report No. CTL/P/1214, submitted to WHO by ICI).

REYNOLDS, L.F. (1984) *Cyhalothrin: Determination of acute toxicity to Bluegill sunfish* (Lepomis machrochirus) (Unpublished proprietary report No. BL/B/2514, submitted to WHO by ICI).

RICHOLD, M., ALLEN, J.A., WILLIAMS, A., & RANSOME, S.J. (1981) *Cell transformation test for potential carcinogenicity of Y00102/010/005 (cyhalothrin (PP563))* (Unpublished proprietary report of the Huntingdon Research Centre No. 391(B)/80948, submitted to WHO by ICI).

ROBERTS, N.L. & FAIRLEY, C. (1981) *The acute oral toxicity (LD_{50}) of cyhalothrin to the Mallard duck* (Unpublished proprietary report of the Huntingdon Research Centre No. 373WL/801024, submitted to WHO by ICI).

ROBERTS, N.L. & FAIRLEY, C. (1984) *The acute oral toxicity (LD_{50}) of PP321 to the Mallard duck* (Unpublished proprietary report of the Huntingdon Research Centre No. 438BT/831011, submitted to WHO by ICI).

ROBERTS, N.L., FAIRLEY, C., & WOODHOUSE, R.N. (1981a) *The subacute dietary toxicity (LC_{50}) of cyhalothrin to the Mallard duck* (Unpublished proprietary report of the Huntingdon Research Centre No. 377WL/8120, submitted to WHO by ICI).

ROBERTS, N.L., FAIRLEY, C., & WOODHOUSE, R.N. (1981b) *The subacute dietary toxicity (LC_{50}) of cyhalothrin to the Bobwhite quail* (Unpublished proprietary report of the Huntingdon Research Centre No. 378WL/8179, submitted to WHO by ICI).

ROBERTS, N.L., FAIRLEY, C., HAKIN, B., PRENTICE, D.E., & WIGHT, D.G.D. (1982) *The acute oral toxicity (LD_{50}) and neurotoxic effects of cyhalothrin to the domestic hen* (Unpublished proprietary report of the Huntingdon Research Centre No. ICI/374 NT/81742, submitted to WHO by ICI).

ROBERTS, N.L., FAIRLEY, C., ANDERSON, A., & DAWE, I.S. (1985a) *The subacute dietary toxicity of PP321 to the Mallard duck* (Unpublished proprietary report of the Huntingdon Research Centre No. ISN 46BT/85171, submitted to WHO by ICI).

ROBERTS, N.L., FAIRLEY, C., ANDERSON, A., & DAWE, I.S. (1985b) *The subacute toxicity of PP321 to the Bobwhite quail* (Unpublished proprietary report of the Huntingdon Research Centre No. ISN 45BT/841287, submitted to WHO by ICI).

RUIGT, G.S.F. & VAN DEN BERCKEN, J. (1986) Action of pyrethroids on a nerve muscle preparation of the clawed frog, *Xenopus laevis*. *Pestic. Biochem. Physiol.*, 25: 176-187.

SAPIETS, A. (1984a) *Cyhalothrin: Storage stability of the residue on deep frozen apple, cabbage and soil samples* (Unpublished proprietary report No. M3843B, submitted to WHO by ICI).

SAPIETS, A. (1984b) *The determination of residues of PP321 in crops. A gas-liquid chromatographic method using an internal standard* (Unpublished proprietary residue analytical method No. PPRAM 81, submitted to WHO by ICI).

SAPIETS, A. (1984c) *The determination of residues of cyhalothrin metabolites in crops. A gas-liquid chromatographic method* (Unpublished proprietary residue analytical method No. PPRAM 74, submitted to WHO by ICI).

SAPIETS, A. (1985a) *The determination of residues of cyhalothrin in crops. A gas-liquid chromatographic method using an internal standard* (Unpublished proprietary residue analytical method No. PPRAM 70, submitted to WHO by ICI).

SAPIETS, A. (1985b) *The determination of residues of cyhalothrin in water. A gas-liquid chromatographic method using an internal standard* (Unpublished proprietary residue analytical method No. PPRAM 69, submitted to WHO by ICI).

SAPIETS, A. (1985c) *PP321: Residue transfer study with dairy cows fed on a diet containing the insecticide* (Unpublished proprietary report No. M3936B, submitted to WHO by ICI).

SAPIETS, A. (1986a) *The determination of residues of PP321 in products of animal origin. A GLC method using an internal standard* (Unpublished proprietary residue analytical method No. PPRAM 86/1, submitted to WHO by ICI).

SAPIETS, A. (1986b) *The determination of residues of PP321 in soil. A GLC method using an internal standard* (Unpublished proprietary residue analytical method No. PPRAM 93, submitted to WHO by ICI).

SAPIETS, A., SWAINE, H., & TANDY, M.J. (1984) In: Zweig, G. & Sherma, J., ed. *Cypermethrin (Chapter 2). Analytical methods for pesticides and plant growth regulators: Vol XIII, Synthetic pyrethroids and other pesticides,* New York, London, San Francisco, Academic Press.

SHELDON, T., RICHARDSON, C.R., SHAW, J., & BARBER, G. (1984) *An evaluation of PP321 in the mouse micronucleus test* (Unpublished proprietary report No. CTL/P/1090, submitted to WHO by ICI).

SHELDON, T., HOWARD, C.A., & RICHARDSON, C.R. (1985) *PP321: A cytogenetic study in human lymphocytes* in vitro (Unpublished proprietary report No. CTL/P/1333, submitted to WHO by ICI).

SMART, L.E. & STEVENSON, J.H. (1982) Laboratory estimation of toxicity of pyrethroid insecticides to honeybees: Relevance to hazard in the field. *Bee World,* **63**(4): 150-152.

SOUTHWOOD, J. (1984) *PP321: Acute oral toxicity to the mouse* (Unpublished proprietary report No. CTL/P/1066, submitted to WHO by ICI).

SOUTHWOOD, J. (1985) *PP321: Acute oral toxicity studies* (Unpublished report No. CTL/P/1102, submitted to WHO by ICI).

STEVENS, J.E.B. & BEWICK, D.W. (1985) *PP563 and PP321: Leaching of PP563 and PP321 and their degradation products in soil columns* (Unpublished proprietary report No. RJ0408B, submitted to WHO by ICI).

TAKEDA CHEMICAL CO. LTD (1979) *Test result of fish toxicity of PP-563* (Unpublished proprietary report, submitted to WHO by ICI).

THOMPSON, R.S. (1985) *PP321: Determination of acute toxicity to Mysid shrimps* (Mysidopsis bahia) (Unpublished proprietary report No. BL/B/2635, submitted to WHO by ICI).

THOMPSON, R.S. & WILLIAMS, T.D. (1985) *PP321: Toxicity to the green alga* Selenastrum capricornutum (Unpublished proprietary report No. BL/B2584, submitted to WHO by ICI).

TINSON, D.J., BANHAM, P.D., CHART, I.S., GORE, C.W., PRATT, I., SCALES, M.D.C., & WEIGHT, T.M. (1984) *PP563: 28-day feeding study in rats. Summary report* (Unpublished proprietary report No. CTL/P/1056, submitted to WHO by ICI).

TRUEMAN, R.W. (1981) *Cyhalothrin: Results from the Salmonella reverse mutation assay* (Unpublished proprietary report No. CTL/P/665, submitted to WHO by ICI).

VAN DEN BERCKEN, J. (1977) The action of allethrin on the peripheral nervous system of the frog. *Pestic. Sci.*, **8**: 692-699.

VAN DEN BERCKEN, J. & VIJVERBERG, H.P.M. (1980) Voltage clamp studies on the effects of allethrin and DDT on the sodium channels in frog myelinated nerve membrane. In: *Insect neurobiology and pesticide action*, London, Society of Chemical Industry, pp. 79-85.

VAN DEN BERCKEN, J., AKKERMANS, L.M.A., & VAN DER ZALM, J.M. (1973) DDT-like action of allethrin in the sensory nervous system of *Xenopus laevis*. *Eur. J. Pharmacol.*, **21**: 95-106.

VAN DEN BERCKEN, J., KROESE, A.B.A., & AKKERMANS, L.M.A. (1979) Effects of insecticides on the sensory nervous system. In: Narashashi, T., ed. *Neurotoxicology of insecticides and pheromones*, New York, London, Plenum Publishing Corporation, pp. 183-210.

VERSCHOYLE, R.D. & ALDRIDGE, W.N. (1980) Structure-activity relationships of some pyrethroids in rats. *Arch. Toxicol.*, **45**: 325-329.

VIJVERBERG, H.P.M. & VAN DEN BERCKEN, J. (1979) Frequency-dependent effects of the pyrethroid insecticide decamethrin in frog myelinated nerve fibres. *Eur. J. Pharmacol.*, **58**: 501-504.

VIJVERBERG, H.P.M. & VAN DEN BERCKEN, J. (1982) Action of pyrethroid insecticides on the vertebrate nervous system. *Neuropathol. appl. Neurobiol.*, **8**: 421-440.

VIJVERBERG, H.P.M., RUIGT, G.S.F., & VAN DEN BERCKEN, J. (1982a) Structure-related effects of pyrethroid insecticides on the lateral-line sense organ and on peripheral nerves of the clawed frog, *Xenopus laevis*. *Pestic. Biochem. Physiol.*, **18**: 315-324.

VIJVERBERG, H.P.M., VAN DER ZALM, J.M., & VAN DEN BERCKEN, J. (1982b) Similar mode of action of pyrethroids and DDT on sodium channel gating in myelinated nerves. *Nature (Lond.)*, **295**: 601-603.

VIJVERBERG, H.P.M., VAN DER ZALM, J.M., VAN KLEEF, R.G.D.M., & VAN DEN BERCKEN, J. (1983) Temperature- and structure-dependent interaction of pyrethroids with the sodium channels in the frog node of Ranvier. *Biochem. Biophys. Acta*, **728**: 73-82.

WHO (1979) *Safe use of pesticides. Third report of the WHO Expert Committee on Vector Biology and Control*, Geneva, World Health Organization (WHO Technical Report Series, No. 634).

WILLIAMS, T.D. & THOMPSON, R.S. (1981) *Determination of the acute toxicity of cyhalothrin (PP563) to* Daphnia magna (Unpublished proprietary report No. BL/B/2114, submitted to WHO by ICI).

WOUTERS, W. & VAN DEN BERCKEN, J. (1978) Action of pyrethroids. *Gen. Pharmacol.*, **9**: 387-398.

YAMAUCHI, F., SHIGEOKA, T., YAMAGATA, T., & SAITO, H. (1984a) *PP563 (cyhalothrin): Accumulation in fish (carp) in a flow-through water system* (Unpublished proprietary report of MITES No. 58-367, submitted to WHO by ICI).

YAMAUCHI, F., SHIGEOKA, T., YAMAGATA, T., & SATO, Y. (1984b) *PP563 (cyhalothrin) formulation (5% WP): Acute toxicity to carp* (Unpublished proprietary report of MITES No. 58-367, submitted to WHO by ICI).

YAMAUCHI, F., SHIGEOKA, T., YAMAGATA, T., & SATO, Y. (1984c) *PP563 (cyhalothrin): Toxicity to daphnia and fish (carp) in the presence and absence of soil* (Unpublished proprietary report of MITES No. 58-367, submitted to WHO by ICI).

YAMAUCHI, F., SHIGEOKA, T., YAMAGATA, T., & SATO, Y. (1984d) *PP563 (cyhalothrin) formulation (5% WP): Acute toxicity to daphnia* (Unpublished proprietary report of MITES No. 58-367, submitted to WHO by ICI).

APPENDIX

On the basis of electrophysiological studies with peripheral nerve preparations of frogs *(Xenopus laevis; Rana temporaria,* and *Rana escuelenta),* it is possible to distinguish between 2 classes of pyrethroid insecticides: (Type I and Type II). A similar distinction between these 2 classes of pyrethroids has been made on the basis of the symptoms of toxicity in mammals and insects (Van den Bercken et al., 1979; WHO, 1979; Verschoyle & Aldridge, 1980; Glickman & Casida, 1982; Lawrence & Casida, 1982). The same distinction was found in studies on cockroaches (Gammon et al., 1981).

Based on the binding assay on the gamma-aminobutyric acid (GABA) receptor-ionophore complex, synthetic pyrethroids can also be classified into two types: the α-cyano-3-phenoxybenzyl pyrethroids and the non-cyano pyrethroids (Gammon et al., 1982; Gammon & Casida, 1983; Lawrence & Casida, 1983; Lawrence et al., 1985).

Pyrethroids that do not contain an α-cyano group (allethrin, d-phenothrin, permethrin, tetramethrin, cismethrin, and bioresmethrin) (Type I: T-syndrome)

The pyrethroids that do not contain an α-cyano group give rise to pronounced repetitive activity in sense organs and in sensory nerve fibres (Van den Bercken et al., 1973). At room temperature, this repetitive activity usually consists of trains of 3-10 impulses and occasionally up to 25 impulses. Train duration is between 10 and 5 milliseconds.

These compounds also induce pronounced repetitive firing of the presynaptic motor nerve terminal in the neuromuscular junction (Van den Bercken, 1977). There was no significant effect of the insecticide on neurotransmitter release or on the sensitivity of the subsynaptic membrane, nor on the muscle fibre membrane. Presynaptic repetitive firing was also observed in the sympathetic ganglion treated with these pyrethroids.

In the lateral-line sense organ and in the motor nerve terminal, but not in the cutaneous touch receptor or in sensory nerve fibres, the pyrethroid-induced repetitive activity increases dramatically as the temperature is lowered, and a decrease of 5 °C in temperature may cause a more than 3-fold increase in the number of repetitive impulses per train. This effect is easily reversed by raising the temperature. The origin of this "negative temperature coefficient" is not clear (Vijverberg et al., 1983).

Synthetic pyrethroids act directly on the axon through interference with the sodium channel gating mechanism that underlies the generation and conduction of each nerve impulse. The transitional state of the sodium channel is controlled by 2 separately acting gating mechanisms, referred to as the activation gate and the inactivation gate. Since pyrethroids only appear to affect the sodium current during depolarization, the rapid opening of the activation gate and the slow closing of the inactivation gate proceed normally. However, once the sodium channel is open, the activation gate is restrained in the open position by the pyrethroid molecule. While all pyrethroids have essentially the same basic mechanism of action, however, the rate of relaxation differs substantially for the various pyrethroids (Flannigan & Tucker, 1985).

In the isolated node of Ranvier, allethrin causes prolongation of the transient increase in sodium permeability of the nerve membrane during excitation (Van den Bercken & Vijverberg, 1980). Evidence so far available indicates that allethrin selectively slows down the closing of the activation gate of a fraction of the sodium channels that open during depolarization of the membrane. The time constant of closing of the activation gate in the allethrin-affected channels is about 100 milliseconds compared with less than 100 microseconds in the normal sodium channel, i.e., it is slowed down by a factor of more than 100. This results in a marked prolongation of the sodium current across the nerve membrane during excitation, and this prolonged sodium current is directly responsible for the repetitive activity induced by allethrin (Vijverberg et al., 1983).

The effects of cismethrin on synaptic transmission in the frog neuromuscular junction, as reported by Evans (1976), are almost identical to those of allethrin, i.e., presynaptic repetitive firing, and no significant effects on transmitter release or on the subsynaptic membrane.

Interestingly, the action of these pyrethroids closely resembles that of the insecticide DDT in the peripheral nervous system of the frog. DDT also causes pronounced repetitive activity in sense organs, in sensory nerve fibres, and in motor nerve terminals, due to a prolongation of the transient increase in sodium permeability of the nerve membrane during excitation. Recently, it was demonstrated that allethrin and DDT have essentially the same effect on sodium channels in frog myelinated nerve membrane. Both compounds slow down the rate of closing of a fraction of the sodium channels that open on depolarization of the membrane (Van den Bercken et al., 1973, 1979; Vijverberg et al., 1982b).

In the electrophysiological experiments using giant axons of cray-fish, the type I pyrethroids and DDT analogues retain sodium channels in a modified open state only intermittently, cause large depolarizing after-potentials, and evoke repetitive firing with minimal effect on the resting potential (Lund & Narahashi, 1983).

These results strongly suggest that permethrin and cismethrin, like allethrin, primarily affect the sodium channels in the nerve membrane and cause a prolongation of the transient increase in sodium permeability of the membrane during excitation.

The effects of pyrethroids on end-plate and muscle action potentials were studied in the pectoralis nerve-muscle preparation of the clawed frog *(Xenopus laevis)*. Type I pyrethroids (allethrin, cismethrin, bioresmethrin, and 1R, *cis*-phenothrin) caused moderate presynaptic repetitive activity, resulting in the occurrence of multiple end-plate potentials (Ruigt & Van den Bercken, 1986).

Pyrethroids with an α-cyano group on the 3-phenoxybenzyl alcohol (deltamethrin, cypermethrin, fenvalerate, and fenpropanate) (Type II: CS-syndrome)

The pyrethroids with an α-cyano group cause an intense repetitive activity in the lateral line organ in the form of long-lasting trains of impulses (Vijverberg et al., 1982a). Such a train may last for up to 1 min and contains thousands of impulses. The duration of the trains and the number of impulses per train increase markedly on lowering the temperature. Cypermethrin does not cause repetitive activity in myelinated nerve fibres. Instead, this pyrethroid causes a frequency-dependant depression of the nervous impulse, brought about by a progressive depolarization of the nerve membrane as a result of the summation of depolarizing after-potentials during train stimulation (Vijverberg & Van den Bercken, 1979; Vijverberg et al., 1983).

In the isolated node of Ranvier, cypermethrin, like allethrin, specifically affects the sodium channels of the nerve membrane and causes a long-lasting prolongation of the transient increase in sodium permeability during excitation, presumably by slowing down the closing of the activation gate of the sodium channel (Vijverberg & Van den Bercken, 1979; Vijverberg et al., 1983). The time constant of closing of the activation gate in the cypermethrin-affected channels is prolonged to more than 100 milliseconds. Apparently, the amplitude of the prolonged sodium current after cypermethrin is too small to induce repetitive activity in nerve fibres, but is sufficient to cause the long-lasting repetitive firing in the lateral-line sense organ.

These results suggest that α-cyano pyrethroids primarily affect the sodium channels in the nerve membrane and cause a long-lasting prolongation of the transient increase in sodium permeability of the membrane during excitation.

In the electrophysiological experiments using giant axons of cray-fish, the Type II pyrethroids retain sodium channels in a modified continuous open state persistently, depolarize the membrane, and block the action potential without causing repetitive firing (Lund & Narahashi, 1983).

Diazepam, which facilitates GABA reaction, delayed the onset of action of deltamethrin and fenvalerate, but not permethrin and allethrin, in both the mouse and cockroach. Possible mechanisms of the Type II pyrethroid syndrome include action at the GABA receptor complex or a closely linked class of neuroreceptor (Gammon et al., 1982).

The Type II syndrome of intracerebrally administered pyrethroids closely approximates that of the convulsant picrotoxin (PTX). Deltamethrin inhibits the binding of [^{3}H]-dihydropicrotoxin to rat brain synaptic membranes, whereas the non-toxic R epimer of deltamethrin is inactive. These findings suggest a possible relation between the Type II pyrethroid action and the GABA receptor complex. The stereospecific correlation between the toxicity of Type II pyrethroids and their potency to inhibit the [^{35}S]-TBPS binding was established using a radioligand, [^{35}S]-*t*-butylbicyclophosphorothionate [^{35}S]-TBPS.

Studies with 37 pyrethroids revealed an absolute correlation, without any false positive or negative, between mouse intracerebral toxicity and *in vitro* inhibition: all toxic cyano compounds including deltamethrin, 1R,*cis*-cypermethrin, 1R,*trans*-cypermethrin, and [2S,α]-fenvalerate were inhibitors, but their non-toxic stereoisomers were not; non-cyano pyrethroids were much less potent or were inactive (Lawrence & Casida, 1983).

In the [^{35}S]-TBPS and [^{3}H]-Ro 5-4864 (a convulsant benzodiazepine radioligand) binding assay, the inhibitory potencies of pyrethroids were closely related to their mammalian toxicities. The most toxic pyrethroids of Type II were the most potent inhibitors of [^{3}H]-Ro 5-4864 specific binding to rat brain membranes. The [^{3}H]-dihydro-picrotoxin and [^{35}S]-TBPS binding studies with pyrethroids strongly indicated that Type II effects of pyrethroids are mediated, at least in part, through an interaction with a GABA-regulated chloride ionophore-associated binding site. Moreover, studies with [^{3}H]-Ro 5-4864 support this hypothesis and, in addition, indicate that the pyrethroid-binding site may be very closely related to the convulsant benzodiazepine site of action (Lawrence et al., 1985).

The Type II pyrethroids (deltamethrin, 1R, *cis*-cypermethrin and [2S, αS]-fenvalerate) increased the input resistance of crayfish claw opener muscle fibres bathed in GABA. In contrast, two non-insecticidal stereoisomers and Type I pyrethroids (permethrin, resmethrin, allethrin) were inactive. Therefore, cyanophenoxybenzyl pyrethroids appear to act on the GABA receptor-ionophore complex (Gammon & Casida, 1983).

The effects of pyrethroids on end-plate and muscle action potentials were studied in the pectoralis nerve-muscle preparation of the clawed frog *(Xenopus laevis)*. Type II pyrethroids (cypermethrin and deltamethrin) induced trains of repetitive muscle action potentials without presynaptic repetitive activity. However, an intermediate group of pyrethroids (1R-permethrin, cyphenothrin, and fenvalerate) caused both types of effect. Thus, in muscle or nerve membrane the pyrethroid induced repetitive activities due to a prolongation of the sodium current. But no clear distinction was observed between non-cyano and α-cyano pyrethroids (Ruigt & Van den Bercken, 1986).

Appraisal

In summary, the results strongly suggest that the primary target site of pyrethroid insecticides in the vertebrate nervous system is the sodium channel in the nerve membrane. Pyrethroids without an α-cyano group (allethrin, d-phenothrin, permethrin, and cismethrin) cause a moderate prolongation of the transient increase in sodium permeability of the nerve membrane during excitation. This results in relatively short trains of repetitive nerve impulses in sense organs, sensory (afferent) nerve fibres, and, in effect, nerve terminals. On the other hand, the α-cyano pyrethroids cause a long-lasting prolongation of the transient increase in sodium permeability of the nerve membrane during excitation. This results in long-lasting trains of repetitive impulses in sense organs and a frequency-dependent depression of the nerve impulse in nerve fibres. The difference in effects between permethrin and cypermethrin, which have identical molecular structures except for the presence of an α-cyano group on the phenoxybenzyl alcohol, indicates that it is this α-cyano group that is responsible for the long-lasting prolongation of the sodium permeability.

Since the mechanisms responsible for nerve impulse generation and conduction are basically the same throughout the entire nervous system, pyrethroids may also induce repetitive activity in various parts of the brain. The difference in symptoms of poisoning by α-cyano pyrethroids, compared with the classical pyrethroids, is not necessarily due to an exclusive central site of action. It may be related to the long-lasting repetitive activity in sense organs and possibly in other parts of the nervous system, which, in a more advance state of poisoning, may be accompanied by a frequency-dependent depression of the nervous impulse.

Pyrethroids also cause pronounced repetitive activity and a prolongation of the transient increase in sodium permeability of the nerve membrane in insects and other invertebrates. Available information indicates that the sodium channel in the nerve membrane is also the most important target site of pyrethroids in the invertebrate nervous system (Wouters & Van den Bercken, 1978; WHO, 1979).

Because of the universal character of the processes underlying nerve excitability, the action of pyrethroids should not be considered restricted to particular animal species, or to a certain region of the nervous system. Although it has been established that sense organs and nerve endings are the most vulnerable to the action of pyrethroids, the ultimate lesion that causes death will depend on the animal species, environmental conditions, and on the chemical structure and physical characteristics of the pyrethroid molecule (Vijverberg & Van den Bercken, 1982).

RESUME, EVALUATION, CONCLUSIONS, ET RECOMMANDATIONS

1. Résumé et évaluation

1.1 Identité, propriétés physiques et chimiques, méthodes d'analyse

La cyhalothrine s'obtient en estérifiant l'acide (chloro-2 trifluoro-3,3,3 propényl-1)-3 diméthyl-2,2 cyclopropanecarboxylique, par l'alcool α-cyanophénoxy-3 benzylique et elle consiste en un mélange de quatre stéréoisomères formant deux paires d'énantiomères. La lambda-cyhalothrine est l'une de ces paires d'énantiomères et constitue la forme la plus active biologiquement.

La cyhalothrine de qualité technique est un liquide visqueux d'un jaune brunâtre (point de fusion environ 10 °C) qui contient plus de 90% de matière active. Elle est constituée de quatre isomères cis dans la proportion de 1:1:1:1. Elle est insoluble dans l'eau mais soluble dans divers solvants organiques, en particulier les hydrocarbures aliphatiques et aromatiques. Elle est stable à la lumière et à la chaleur et possède une faible tension de vapeur.

La lambda-cyhalothrine technique est un solide beige (point de fusion 49,2 °C) contenant plus de 90% de matière active. Le rapport des énantiomères (Z) (1R, 3R) de l'ester S aux énantiomères (Z) (1S, 3S) de l'ester R est de 1:1. Peu soluble dans l'eau, ce produit est soluble dans divers solvants organiques et possède une faible tension de vapeur. La cyhalothrine et la lambda-cyhalothrine sont rapidement hydrolysées en milieu alcalin mais ne subissent aucune hydrolyse en milieu neutre ou acide.

On dispose de méthodes confirmées pour la recherche et le dosage des résidus de cyhalothrine et de lambda-cyhalothrine ainsi que pour l'analyse des prélèvements effectués dans l'environnement (limite inférieure de détection: 0,005 mg/kg).

1.2 Production et usage

La cyhalothrine a été mise au point en 1977. On l'utilise principalement pour détruire diverses espèces nuisibles en santé publique et santé publique vétérinaire ainsi qu'en agriculture contre les ravageurs des fruits à pépins. La lambda-cyhalothrine est utilisée essentiellement en agriculture pour la protection des récoltes les plus variées et fait actuellement l'objet d'une mise au point en vue d'être utilisée en santé publique.

On ne dispose d'aucune donnée sur les quantités produites.

1.3 Exposition humaine

Les résidus dans les produits alimentaires, par suite du traitement des récoltes par la cyhalothrine et la lambda-cyhalothrine ainsi que de leur utilisation en médecine vétérinaire sont faibles, généralement inférieurs à 0,2 mg/kg. On ignore quel est l'apport total d'origine alimentaire chez l'homme mais on peut supposer que l'exposition de la population générale par cette voie ne dépasse pas la DJA (0,02 mg/kg de poids corporel).

1.4 Exposition et destinée dans l'environnement

A la surface du sol et en solution aqueuse à pH 5, la lambda-cyhalothrine se décompose sous l'effet du rayonnement solaire avec une demi-vie d'environ 30 jours. Les principaux produits de décomposition sont l'acide (chloro-2 trifluoro-3,3,3 propényl-1)-3 diméthyl-2,2 cyclopropanecarboxylique, l'amide correspondant et l'acide phénoxy-3 benzoïque.

Dans le sol, la dégradation s'effectue principalement par hydroxylation puis rupture de la liaison ester aboutissant à deux produits principaux dont la dégradation se poursuit jusqu'à obtention de dioxyde de carbone. La demi-vie initiale varie de 22 à 82 jours.

La cyhalothrine et la lambda-cyhalothrine sont adsorbées sur les particules du sol et ne se déplacent pas dans l'environnement.

Sur les végétaux, la lambda-cyhalothrine se décompose à vitesse modérée (demi-vie allant jusqu'à 40 jours) de sorte que les résidus sont principalement constitués du composé initial. On trouve également des métabolites en faibles quantités qui résultent d'un certain nombre de réactions d'hydrolyse et d'oxydation.

On ne dispose d'aucune donnée sur les quantités effectivement présentes dans l'environnement mais compte tenu du fait que ce produit est relativement peu utilisé et à doses réduites, ces quantités sont vraisemblablement faibles.

1.5 Absorption, métabolisme, et excrétion

Des études métaboliques ont été effectuées sur des rats, des chiens, des vaches et des chèvres. Chez les rats et les chiens, on a montré que la cyhalothrine administrée par voie orale était bien absorbée, fortement métabolisée, puis éliminée sous forme de conjugués polaires dans les urines. Chez le rat, on a constaté que le taux de cyhalothrine tissulaire diminuait après cessation de l'exposition. Dans les carcasses, les résidus étaient faibles (moins de 5% de la dose au bout de sept jours) et consistaient presque entièrement en cyhalothrine accumulée dans le tissu adipeux. Les résidus présents dans les tissus adipeux étaient éliminés avec une demi-vie de 23 jours.

Après administration par voie orale de cyhalothrine à des vaches en lactation, on a constaté que le produit était rapidement éliminé et qu'un état d'équilibre s'établissait au bout de trois jours entre ingestion et élimination. Vingt-sept pour cent de la dose étaient excrétés dans les urines, 50% dans les matières fécales et 0,8% dans le lait. Les produits retrouvés dans les urines étaient entièrement constitués de métabolites résultant du clivage de l'ester et de leurs conjugués, alors que 60 à 70% des produits marqués au ^{14}C retrouvés dans les matières fécales consistaient en cyhalothrine non métabolisée. Les résidus tissulaires, mesurés 16 heures après l'administration de la dernière dose, étaient faibles, la concentration la plus élevée étant enregistrée dans le tissu adipeux. Les résidus marqués au ^{14}C retrouvés dans le lait et les tissus adipeux étaient presque entièrement constitués de cyhalothrine non métabolisée, à l'exclusion de tout autre composé.

Chez toutes les espèces mammaliennes étudiées, on a constaté que la cyhalothrine subissait une forte métabolisation par clivage de l'ester en acide cyclopropanecarboxylique et acide phénoxy-3 benzoïque et qu'elle était éliminée sous forme de conjugués.

Chez les poissons, les principaux résidus tissulaires consistent en cyhalothrine non métabolisée à côté de quantités plus faibles de produits résultant du clivage de l'ester.

1.6 Effets sur les êtres vivants dans leur milieu naturel

Dans les conditions du laboratoire où la concentration est constante, la cyhalothrine et la lambda-cyhalothrine se révèlent très toxiques pour les poissons et les invertébrés aquatiques. Les valeurs de la CL_{50} à 96 heures pour les poissons vont de 0,2 à 1,3 µg/litre, la CL_{50} à 48 heures pour les invertébrés aquatiques se situant entre 0,008 et 0,04 µg/litre.

En étudiant au laboratoire l'accumulation de la cyhalothrine à concentration constante, on a observé une absorption rapide par les poissons (facteur d'accumulation d'environ 1000 à 2000). Toutefois lorsqu'il y a un sol et des sédiments en suspension, on constate une forte réduction du facteur de bioaccumulation, qui passe à 19 pour les poissons et à 194 pour les daphnies. Lorsqu'on remet les poissons et les daphnies dans de l'eau propre, on constate une diminution rapide des résidus, avec une demi-vie respective de 7 et 1 jours. Il est vraisemblable qu'en utilisation agricole normale, la cyhalothrine et la lambda-cyhalothrine subsistent à faible concentration dans l'eau. Etant donné que ces composés sont rapidement adsorbés et dégradés dans les conditions naturelles, il ne se pose en pratique aucun problème d'accumulation de résidus ni de toxicité vis-à-vis des espèces aquatiques.

La cyhalothrine et la lambda-cyhalothrine sont pratiquement inoffensives pour les oiseaux; la DL_{50} (dose unique) s'est révélée supérieure à 3950 mg/kg pour toutes les espèces étudiées et la CL_{50} alimentaire à cinq jours la plus faible a été de 3948 mg/kg pour des canards sauvages de huit jours qui recevaient de la lambda-cyhalothrine dans leur alimentation.

Dans les conditions du laboratoire, la cyhalothrine et la lambda-cyhalothrine sont toxiques pour les abeilles; la DL_{50} par voie orale est de 0,97 µg de lambda-cyhalothrine par abeille. Toutefois, le risque est probablement moins élevé en pratique étant donné que les formulations actuellement en usage exercent une action répulsive qui empêche les abeilles de butiner sur les récoltes traitées. Lorsque les abeilles se remettent à butiner, on ne constate pas d'augmentation importante de la mortalité.

1.7 Effets sur les animaux d'expérience et les systèmes d'épreuve *in vitro*

La toxicité aiguë par voie orale de la cyhalothrine est modérée chez les rats et les souris et faible chez les cobayes et les lapins (les valeurs de la DL_{50} sont les suivantes: rat, 144-243 mg/kg; souris, 37-62 mg/kg; cobaye, plus de 5000 mg/kg; lapin, plus de 1000 mg/kg). La toxicité aiguë par voie orale de la lambda-cyhalothrine est plus forte que celle de la cyhalothrine (les valeurs de la DL_{50} sont les suivantes: 56-79 mg/kg pour le rat et 20 mg/kg pour la souris). Par voie dermique, on obtient les toxicités suivantes exprimées par la DL_{50}: rat, 200-2000 mg/kg (cyhalothrine), 632-696 mg/kg (lambda-cyhalothrine); lapin, plus de 2000 mg/kg (cyhalothrine). La cyhalothrine et la lambda-cyhalothrine sont des pyréthroïdes du type II avec pour signes cliniques d'intoxication une ataxie, une démarche chancelante et une hyperexcitabilité.

Chez le lapin, la cyhalothrine est modérément irritante pour l'oeil et la lambda-cyhalothrine peu irritante; les deux composés sont légèrement irritants pour la peau. La cyhalothrine n'est pas irritante pour la peau chez le rat. Toutefois elle provoque une sensibilisation cutanée modérée chez le cobaye. La lambda-cyhalothrine n'a pas d'action sensibilisatrice sur la peau.

Lors d'une étude d'alimentation de 90 jours au cours de laquelle des rats ont reçu de la cyhalothrine à des doses allant jusqu'à 250 mg/kg de nourriture, on a observé une réduction du gain de poids chez les mâles à la dose la plus forte. Des effets marginaux sur la valeur moyenne de l'hématocrite ont été enregistrés chez certains des groupes traités ainsi que quelques modifications au niveau du foie que l'on a considérées comme résultant d'une réaction d'adaptation. Lors d'une étude de 90 jours au cours de laquelle des rats ont reçu dans leur alimentation de la lambda-cyhalothrine à des doses allant jusqu'à 250 mg/kg de nourriture, on a observé une réduction du gain de poids chez les deux sexes à la dose la plus forte. On a observé un certain nombre d'effets sur le chimisme sanguin ainsi que des effets hépatiques analogues à ceux qui avaient été observés avec la cyhalothrine. La dose sans effet observable était de 50 mg/kg de nourriture.

Lors d'une étude de 26 semaines au cours de laquelle de la cyhalothrine a été administrée par voie orale à des chiens à des doses quotidiennes allant jusqu'à 10 mg/kg de poids corporel, on a observé des signes d'intoxication de type pyréthroïde à la dose la plus forte. La dose sans effet observable se situait à 2,5 mg/kg de poids corporel. Une étude du même genre a été menée sur d'autres chiens avec administration pendant 52 semaines de 3,5 mg de lambda-cyhalothrine par kg de poids corporel et par jour. Des signes cliniques d'intoxication de type pyréthroïde (signes neurologiques) ont été observés chez tous les animaux à la dose quotidienne de 3,5 mg/kg de poids corporel. La dose sans effet observable se situait à 0,5 mg/kg de poids corporel par jour.

Lors d'une étude de toxicité cutanée de 21 jours pratiquée sur des lapins au moyen d'une solution de cyhalothrine dans le polyéthylène-glycol à des doses quotidiennes allant jusqu'à 1000 mg/kg de poids corporel, on a constaté des signes cliniques d'intoxication chez certains des animaux à la dose la plus forte. Dans tous les groupes, y compris les témoins, on a observé une irritation cutanée légère à sévère.

Deux études toxicologiques de 104 semaines ont été consacrées à la cyhalothrine, l'une sur des rats et l'autre sur des souris. L'étude sur le rat n'a révélé aucun effet oncogène à des doses allant jusqu'à 250 mg/kg de nourriture (dose la plus forte étudiée). La dose sans effet observable en ce qui concerne la toxicité générale était de 50 mg/kg de nourriture (1,8 mg/kg de poids corporel par jour). On a relevé une diminution du gain de poids corporel chez les deux sexes à la dose de 250 mg/kg de nourriture. Aucun effet oncogène n'a été observé chez la souris à des doses allant jusqu'à 500 mg/kg de nourriture (dose la plus forte étudiée). Les signes cliniques d'une intoxication de type pyréthroïde ont été observés aux doses de 100 et 500 mg/kg de nourriture, avec réduction du gain de poids corporel à cette dernière dose.

En ce qui concerne la toxicité générale, la dose sans effet observable était de 20 mg/kg de nourriture (1,9 mg/kg de poids corporel par jour). Aucun signe histologique de lésion du système nerveux n'a été observé dans l'une ou l'autre de ces deux études.

Lors d'une série d'épreuves *in vivo* et *in vitro* visant à déceler des mutations géniques, des lésions chromosomiques et autres effets génotoxiques, on n'a observé aucun effet de ce type imputable à la cyhalothrine ou à la lambda-cyhalothrine. Administrée par voie orale à des rats et à des lapins au cours de la période cruciale de l'organogénèse, la cyhalothrine ne s'est révélée ni embryotoxique ni tératogène à des doses quotidiennes qui étaient toxiques pour la mère (15 mg/kg pour les rats et 30 mg/kg pour les lapins, c'est-à-dire les deux doses les plus fortes étudiées).

Lors d'une étude de reproduction portant sur trois générations, des rats ont reçu de la cyhalothrine dans leur alimentation à des doses allant jusqu'à 100 mg/kg de nourriture. A la dose de 100 mg/kg de nourriture on a observé une légère diminution de la taille des portées et une réduction peu importante du gain de poids. En ce qui concerne les effets sur la reproduction, la dose sans effet observable était de 30 mg/kg de nourriture.

1.8 Effets sur l'homme

Aucun cas d'intoxication accidentelle n'a été décrit.

Des sensations subjectives au niveau de la face ont été ressenties lors de la fabrication, de la formulation, du travail de laboratoire et de l'utilisation sur le terrain. Cet effet ne dure en général que quelques heures mais il arrive qu'il se prolonge jusqu'à 72 heures après l'exposition; l'examen médical n'a pas révélé d'anomalies neurologiques.

Ces sensations cutanées subjectives au niveau de la face, qui sont ressenties par les personnes qui manipulent de la cyhalothrine ou de la lambda-cyhalothrine sont, semble-t-il, provoquées par l'excitation répétée des terminaisons nerveuses de la peau. On peut les considérer comme un signal d'alarme qui indique une surexposition de l'épiderme.

Rien n'indique que la cyhalothrine et la lambda-cyhalothrine puissent avoir des effets nocifs pour l'homme lorsqu'on les utilise dans les conditions et aux doses qui sont recommandées actuellement.

2. Conclusions

a) *Population générale:* l'exposition de la population générale à la cyhalothrine et à la lambda-cyhalothrine est vraisemblablement très faible et ne présente probablement aucun danger lorsque ces produits sont utilisés conformément aux recommandations.

b) *Exposition professionnelle:* moyennant de bonnes méthodes de travail, des mesures d'hygiène et pour peu que l'on respecte les précautions nécessaires, la cyhalothrine et la lambda-cyhalothrine ne présentent vraisemblablement aucun danger pour les personnes exposées de par leur profession.

c) *Environnement:* il ne semble pas que la cyhalothrine, la lambda-cyhalothrine ou leurs produits de dégradation puissent atteindre des concentrations nocives pour l'environnement lorsqu'elles sont utilisées aux doses recommandées. Dans les conditions du laboratoire, la cyhalothrine et la lambda-cyhalothrine sont très toxiques pour les poissons, les arthropodes aquatiques et les abeilles. Toutefois, en pratique, il ne semble pas qu'il puisse se produire d'effets nocifs durables, lorsque ces insecticides sont utilisés conformément aux recommandations.

3. Recommandations

Lorsque ces insecticides sont utilisés conformément aux recommandations, leurs concentrations dans les denrées alimentaires doivent être très faibles, toutefois il serait bon de le confirmer en soumettant la cyhalothrine et la lambda-cyhalothrine à une surveillance.

La cyhalothrine et la lambda-cyhalothrine sont utilisées depuis des années et seuls des effets passagers ont été observés lors d'expositions professionnelles; toutefois il faut continuer à surveiller l'exposition humaine.

RESUMEN, EVALUACION, CONCLUSIONES Y RECOMENDACIONES

1. Resumen y evaluación

1.1 Identidad, propiedades físicas y químicas, y métodos analíticos

La cihalotrina se obtiene esterificando ácido 3-(2-cloro-3,3,3-trifluoroprop-1-enil)-2,2-dimetilciclopropanocarboxílico con alcohol α-ciano-3-fenoxibencílico y se compone de una mezcla de cuatro estereoisómeros. La lambda-cihalotrina se compone de un par enantiomérico de isómeros y es la forma más activa biológicamente.

La cihalotrina de calidad técnica es un líquido viscoso, de color entre amarillo y marrón (punto de fusión: aproximadamente 10 °C), que contiene más del 90% de material activo. Está compuesta por cuatro isómeros cis en proporción 1:1:1:1. Aunque es insoluble en el agua, es soluble en toda una gama de disolventes orgánicos como los hidrocarburos alifáticos y aromáticos. Es estable respecto de la luz y la temperatura y tiene una baja tensión de vapor.

La lambda-cihalotrina de calidad técnica es un sólido de color café con leche (punto de fusión: 49,2 °C) que contiene más del 90% de material activo. La razón enantiomérica del *(Z), (1R, 3R)*, S-éster y el *(Z), (1S, 3S)*, R-éster es 1:1. Es apenas soluble en el agua pero es soluble en toda una gama de disolventes orgánicos y tiene una baja tensión de vapor. Tanto la cihalotrina como la lambda-cihalotrina se hidrolizan rápidamente en medio alcalino pero no en medio neutro o ácido.

Existen métodos bien establecidos para analizar la cihalotrina y la lambda-cihalotrina presentes en residuos y en el medio ambiente (la concentración detectable mínima es 0,005 mg/kg).

1.2 Producción y utilización

La cihalotrina comenzó a producirse en 1977. Se utiliza sobre todo para combatir múltiples plagas en salud pública y en veterinaria, pero también se emplea en agricultura contra las plagas que atacan a los pomos. La lambda-cihalotrina se usa principalmente como plaguicida agrícola aplicable a muy diversos cultivos y se está preparando para emplearla en salud pública.

No se dispone de datos sobre los niveles de producción.

1.3 Exposición humana

Los residuos presentes en los alimentos de resultas de la aplicación de cihalotrina y lamba-cihalotrina a los cultivos y en veterinaria son bajos, por lo general inferiores a 0,2 mg/kg. No se dispone de datos sobre la ingesta total en la dieta humana, pero se puede suponer que la exposición dietética de la población general no supera la IDA (0,02 mg/kg de peso corporal).

1.4 Exposición y transformación en el medio ambiente

En la superficie del suelo y en soluciones acuosas con un pH de 5, la lambda-cihalotrina se degrada a la luz del sol con una semivida de unos 30 días. Los principales productos de esa degradación son ácido 3-(2-cloro-3,3,3-trifluoroprop-1-enil)-2,2-dimetilciclopropanocarboxílico, el derivado amídico de la cihalotrina, y ácido 3-fenoxibenzoico.

La degradación en el suelo se produce primordialmente por hidroxilación seguida de la ruptura del enlace éster para dar lugar a dos principales productos de degradación, que siguen degradándose hasta convertirse en bióxido de carbono. Las semividas iniciales oscilan entre 22 y 82 días.

La cihalotrina y la lambda-cihalotrina se adsorben a las partículas del suelo y no son móviles en el medio ambiente.

En las plantas, la lambda-cihalotrina se degrada a un ritmo moderado (semivida de hasta 40 días), por lo que el principal elemento constituyente de los residuos que en ellas se encuentran es por lo común el compuesto inicial. Se hallan también niveles más bajos de metabolitos, resultantes de diversas reacciones hidrolíticas y oxidantes.

No se dispone de datos sobre los niveles efectivos en el medio ambiente, pero dadas la escasa utilización habitual en la actualidad y las reducidas tasas de aplicación, se supone que son bajos.

1.5 Incorporación, metabolismo y excreción

Se han realizado estudios metabólicos en la rata, el perro, la vaca y la cabra. En la rata y el perro se ha demostrado que la cihalotrina administrada por vía oral se absorbe y se metaboliza bien y se elimina en la orina, en forma de conjugados polares. En los tejidos de las ratas, disminuyó la concentración de cihalotrina al interrumpirse la exposición al compuesto. En los cadáveres de las ratas se encontraron niveles reducidos de residuos (< 5% de la dosis a los siete días), que se debían casi totalmente a la cihalotrina contenida en las grasas. Los restos presentes en las grasas se eliminaron con una semivida de 23 días.

La cihalotrina administrada por vía oral a vacas lactantes se eliminó rápidamente, alcanzándose un equilibrio entre la ingestión y la eliminación a los tres días. De la dosis total, el 27% se excretó en la orina, el 50% en las heces, y el 0,8% en la leche. El material presente en la orina estaba compuesto exclusivamente por metabolitos de la disociación de los ésteres y por sus conjugados, mientras que del 60% al 70% del material fecal marcado con [^{14}C] se identificó como cihalotrina no alterada. Dieciséis horas después de la última dosis, los residuos tisulares eran bajos, hallándose las concentraciones más elevadas en las grasas. Los residuos marcados con [^{14}C] presentes en la leche y los tejidos adiposos constaban casi enteramente de cihalotrina no alterada, y no se detectó ningún otro componente.

En todas las especies de mamíferos investigadas, se ha descubierto que la cihalotrina se metaboliza ampliamente de resultas de la ruptura del enlace éster para dar ácido ciclopropanocarboxílico y ácido 3-fenoxibenzoico, y se elimina en forma de conjugados.

En los peces, el principal residuo presente en los tejidos es cihalotrina no alterada y hay niveles más bajos de los productos de la ruptura del éster.

1.6 Efectos en los organismos del medio ambiente

En condiciones de laboratorio con concentraciones tóxicas constantes, la cihalotrina y la lambda-cihalotrina son muy tóxicas para los peces y los invertebrados acuáticos. El valor de las CL_{50} a las 96 horas para los peces oscila entre 0,2 y 1,3 μg/litro, mientras que en el caso de los invertebrados acuáticos los valores de la CL_{50} a las 48 horas van de 0,008 a 0,4 μg/litro.

Los estudios sobre la acumulación realizados en condiciones de laboratorio con concentraciones constantes indican que, en los peces, tiene lugar una rápida incorporación (factor de acumulación aproximado de 1000 a 2000). No obstante, en presencia de suelo y sedimentos en suspensión, los factores de bioacumulación quedan muy reducidos (a 19 en el caso de los peces y a 194 en el caso de los dáfnidos). Cuando se colocó en agua limpia a los peces y dáfnidos expuestos, los residuos disminuyeron rápidamente, con semividas de siete días y un día, respectivamente. Las concentraciones de cihalotrina y lambda-cihalotrina que pueden hallarse en el agua de resultas de su aplicación normal con fines agrícolas serán bajas. Como el compuesto se adsorbe y se degrada rápidamente en condiciones naturales, la acumulación de residuos o la toxicidad de la cihalotrina y la lambda-cihalotrina para las especies acuáticas no plantearán problemas prácticos.

La cihalotrina y la lambda-cihalotrina son prácticamente inocuas para las aves; en todas las especies sometidas a prueba la DL_{50} con una dosis única fue superior a 3950 mg/kg y la CL_{50} dietética más baja en cinco días fue de 3948 mg/kg (lambda-cihalotrina administrada en el alimento a patos silvestres de ocho días de edad).

En condiciones de laboratorio, la cihalotrina y la lambda-cihalotrina son tóxicas para la abeja; la DL_{50} de la lambda-cihalotrina por vía oral es de 0,97 μg/abeja. No obstante, en la práctica, el riesgo es menor puesto que las formas actualmente utilizadas tienen un efecto repelente que hace que las abejas suspendan las actividades de búsqueda en los cultivos tratados. Cuando éstas vuelven a emprenderse, no hay un aumento significativo de la mortalidad de las abejas.

1.7 Efectos en animales de experimentación y en sistemas de prueba *in vitro*

La toxicidad aguda de la cihalotrina administrada por vía oral es moderada para las ratas y los ratones y baja para las cobayas y los conejos (los valores de la DL_{50} son los siguientes: rata: 144-243 mg/kg; ratón: 37-62 mg/kg; cobaya: > 5000 mg/kg; conejo: > 1000 mg/kg). La toxicidad aguda de la lambda-cihalotrina por vía oral es mayor que la de la cihalotrina (los valores de la DL_{50} son: 56-79 mg/kg para la rata y 20 mg/kg para el ratón). La toxicidad por vía cutánea (DL_{50}) alcanza los siguientes valores: rata: 200-2000 mg/kg (cihalotrina), 632-696 mg/kg (lambda-cihalotrina); conejo: > 2000 mg/kg (cihalotrina). La cihalotrina y la lambda-cihalotrina son piretroides de tipo II; entre los signos clínicos figuran la ataxia, el andar vacilante y la hiperexcitabilidad.

En el conejo, la cihalotrina es un irritante ocular moderado y la lambda-cihalotrina un irritante ocular leve; ambos irritan levemente la piel. La cihalotrina no irrita la piel de la rata. Sin embargo, sensibiliza moderadamente la piel de la cobaya. La lambda-cihalotrina no sensibiliza la piel.

En un estudio de alimentación de 90 días en el que se administró cihalotrina a ratas en dosis de hasta 250 mg/kg de alimento, se observó una disminución del aumento del peso corporal en los machos con la dosis de 250 mg. En algunos de los grupos tratados, se señalaron efectos marginales en los volúmenes medios de eritrocitos, así como ciertas alteraciones hepáticas, que se consideraron una respuesta adaptativa. En otro estudio de alimentación de 90 días, en el que se administró lambda-cihalotrina a ratas en dosis de hasta 250 mg/kg de alimento, se observó en ambos sexos una reducción del aumento del peso corporal con la dosis de 250 mg. Se señalaron también algunos efectos en la química clínica, así como efectos hepáticos análogos a los observados con la cihalotrina. El nivel sin efecto observado fue de 50 mg/kg de alimento.

En un estudio de 26 semanas en el que se administraron a perros por vía oral dosis diarias de cihalotrina de hasta 10 mg/kg de peso corporal, se observaron signos de toxicidad por piretroides con la dosis de 10 mg. El nivel sin efecto observado fue de 2,5 mg/kg de peso corporal al día. Se realizó otro estudio similar en el que se administraron a perros, durante 52 semanas, dosis diarias de lambda-cihalotrina de hasta 3,5 mg/kg de peso corporal. En todos los animales que recibieron la dosis de 3,5 mg se observaron signos clínicos de toxicidad por piretroides (signos neurológicos). El nivel sin efecto observado fue de 0,5 mg/kg de peso corporal al día.

En un estudio cutáneo de 21 días con conejos a los que se aplicó cihalotrina en polietilénglicol en dosis diarias de hasta 1000 mg/kg, se observaron en algunos animales signos clínicos de toxicidad con la dosis más alta. En todos los grupos, incluidos los testigos, se señaló irritación de la piel de leve a grave.

Se realizaron dos estudios de alimentación de 104 semanas con cihalotrina, uno con ratas y otro con ratones. En el estudio con ratas, no se observaron efectos oncogénicos con dosis de hasta 250 mg/kg de alimento (la dosis más alta ensayada). En cuanto a la toxicidad sistémica, el nivel sin efecto observado fue de 50 mg/kg de alimento (1,8 mg/kg de peso corporal al día). Con dosis de 250 mg se señaló en ambos sexos una disminución del aumento del peso corporal. En el estudio con ratones, no se observaron efectos oncogénicos con dosis de hasta 500 mg/kg de alimento (la dosis más alta ensayada). Con dosis de 100 y 500 mg/kg de alimento se apreciaron signos clínicos de toxicidad por piretroides y, con dosis de 500 mg, una disminución del aumento del peso corporal. En cuanto a la toxicidad sistémica, el nivel sin efecto observado fue de 20 mg/kg de alimento (1,9 mg/kg de peso corporal al día). En ninguno de los dos estudios se obtuvieron datos histológicos que indicaran la presencia de lesiones del sistema nervioso.

En una serie de pruebas *in vivo* e *in vitro* destinadas a detectar mutaciones génicas, lesiones cromosómicas y otros efectos genotóxicos, se obtuvieron resultados negativos con la cihalotrina y la lambda-cihalotrina. La cihalotrina administrada por vía oral a ratas y conejos durante el periodo de organogénesis principal no resultó embriotóxica ni teratogénica en dosis que provocaron reacciones tóxicas en las madres (15 mg/kg diarios para las ratas y 30 mg/kg diarios para los conejos, en ambos casos los niveles más altos ensayados).

Se realizó un estudio sobre la reproducción en tres generaciones de ratas a las que se administró cihalotrina en dosis de hasta 100 mg/kg de alimento. Con la dosis de 100 mg se observaron pequeñas reducciones del tamaño de las camadas y del aumento de peso. En los aspectos relacionados con la reproducción, el nivel sin efecto observado fue de 30 mg/kg de alimento.

1.8 *Efectos en el ser humano*

No se ha descrito ningún caso de intoxicación accidental.

En las actividades de fabricación, formulación y laboratorio y durante el uso sobre el terreno, se han notificado sensaciones faciales subjetivas. Este efecto sólo suele durar unas horas, pero ocasionalmente persiste hasta 72 horas después de la exposición; el examen médico no ha revelado ninguna anomalía neurológica.

Se cree que las sensaciones cutáneas faciales subjetivas que pueden experimentar las personas que manipulan cihalotrina y lambda-cihalotrina se deben a la repetida estimulación de las terminaciones nerviosas de la piel. Pueden considerarse una señal de alerta que indica que la piel ha sufrido una exposición excesiva.

No hay ninguna indicación de que la cihalotrina y la lambda-cihalotrina, utilizadas en las condiciones y con arreglo a las tasas de aplicación actualmente recomendadas, tengan efectos adversos en los seres humanos.

2. Conclusiones

(a) *Población general:* Se cree que la exposición de la población general a la cihalotrina y la lambda-cihalotrina es muy baja y que no es probable que represente un riesgo en las condiciones de uso recomendadas.

(b) *Exposición ocupacional:* Con prácticas de trabajo, medidas de higiene y precauciones de seguridad adecuadas, es poco probable que la cihalotrina y la lambda-cihalotrina representen un riesgo para las personas ocupacionalmente expuestas.

(c) *Medio ambiente:* No es probable que la cihalotrina y la lambda-cihalotrina o los productos de su degradación alcancen niveles ambientales que puedan producir efectos adversos, si se respetan las tasas de aplicación recomendadas. En condiciones de laboratorio, la cihalotrina y la lambda-cihalotrina son muy tóxicas para los peces, los artrópodos acuáticos y las abejas. No obstante, en la práctica, no es probable que se produzcan efectos adversos duraderos en las condiciones de uso recomendadas.

3. Recomendaciones

Aunque se cree que los niveles dietéticos según el uso recomendado son muy bajos, debe considerarse la posibilidad de confirmar este extremo incluyendo la cihalotrina y la lambda-cihalotrina en estudios de vigilancia.

Pese a que ambas sustancias se llevan utilizando varios años y a que los efectos observados de la exposición ocupacional sólo han sido transitorios, debe continuar la observación de la exposición humana.